~

Privileged Presence

Personal Stories of
Connections in Health Care

Liz Crocker
and
Bev Johnson

~

SECOND EDITION

Bull Publishing Company
Boulder, Colorado

Bull Publishing Company
P.O. Box 1377
Boulder, CO 80306
Phone (800) 676-2855 / Fax (303) 545-6354
www.bullpub.com

Manufactured in the United States of America
Distributed in the United States by
Independent Publishers Group, 814 N. Franklin Street, Chicago, IL 60610

Library of Congress Cataloging-in-Publication Data

Crocker, Liz.
    Privileged presence : personal stories of connections in health care / Liz Crocker
and Bev Johnson. -- Second edition.
        pages cm
    Summary: "Privileged Presence is a collection of more than 50 stories that
capture both the medical and emotional aspects of the health care experience
through tales from those who have been there, and offers powerful messages
about the essential ingredients of "good" health care: respect, compassion,
collaboration, open and honest communication, family involvement, and
flexibility and responsiveness to individuals and their needs. This updated
second edition uses real-world experiences recounted by patients and their
families, nurses, doctors, and other health care professionals to illustrate what
works and what doesn't and what increases or diminishes people's sense of
confidence and well-being"-- Provided by publisher.
    Includes bibliographical references and index.
    ISBN 978-1-936693-69-6 (paperback)
    1. Medical care--Anecdotes. I. Johnson, Beverley H. II. Title.
    RA425.C855 2014
    362.1--dc23
                                                                                2014018696

Interior design and production by Dovetail Publishing Services
Cover design and production by Shannon Bodie, Lightbourne, Inc.

CONTENTS

Contents

Natural Allies: Partnerships in Care 97

More than Words:
Feeling Heard and Being Valued 151

Contents

Contents

Contents

We dedicate this book to our families
who have both grounded us and
provided the encouragement and
inspiration to work with others.

ACKNOWLEDGMENTS

Privileged Presence has come into being because of the generosity of people's spirits, either through their encouragement, their thoughtful comments along the way, or their willingness to share personal stories. Many people suggested sources and contacts; others directly shared their memories, both positive and painful; and some offered constructive feedback and steady support.

On those rare, rare days when we questioned the value of this project, we had important "cheerleaders" who reminded us that so much in health care is positive, yet, at the same time, so much needs to be improved. Often, all we had to do was hear another story to be propelled forward.

The following people are all embedded in the heart and soul of *Privileged Presence*. To each and every one of you, we are grateful beyond words: David Abelson, Marie Abraham, Susan Adair, Alex Aguzzi, Martine Andrews, Richard Antonelli, Catherine Aquino-Russell, Tori Bayless, Hon. Monique Begin, Vicky Bennet, Holly Book, Janet Braunstein, Jane Buss, Carole Carpenter, Linda Clarke, Ellen Cohen, Maureen Connor, Jim Conway, Caren Cramer, Brian Crocker, Catherine Crocker, Suzy Crocker, Colette Deveau, Nancy DiVenere, Nancy Dugas, Kathy Dutton, Susan Edgman-Leviton, Bertha Etter, Sean Farough, Shannon Farough, Wayne Fiander, Marlene Fondrick, Gerri Frager, Margot Gall, Debbie Gillis, Stella Girard, Richard B. Goldbloom, Danny Graham, Jackie Gruzenski, Geri Haight, Kathleen Hipwell, Chuck Hofius, Linda Hofler, Lawrence Horwitz, Stanfield Johnson, Amy Jones, Malori Keller, Donna Koller, Betty Lacas, Judy Lavigniac, Ryan Liebenberg, Fay Lim-Lambie, Linda Larin, Fiona Liston, Beth Lown, Eve McDermott, Sandy McDougall, Kim McInnis, Scott McInnis, Nancy Milford, Heather Mitchell, David Murphy,

Margaret Murphy, Sallie Patel, Sherry Perkins, Ann-Marie Thomas, Kerol Rose, Julie Ann Rosen, Janet Ross, Anna Roth, Michael Rowe, Kelly Roy, Anna Maria Rumble, Saki Santorelli, Juliette Schlucter, Bill Schwab, Will Schwalbe, The Schwartz Center for Compassionate Healthcare, Ann Selinger, Terri L. Shelton, Sue Sheridan, Harriet Shlossberg, Catherine Sloan, Terrell Smith, Perry Spencer, David Spero, Pam Stein, Deborah Stern, Ann-Marie Thomas, Donna Thompson, Ian Thompson, Sue Uteck, Armando Vallin, Debbie Yokoe, Katie Zedible.

Authors' proceeds from the sale of this book are being given to the Institute for Patient- and Family-Centered Care in Bethesda, Maryland.

Foreword

Is *Privileged Presence* Making a Difference?

When *Privileged Presence* was first published in 2006, we hoped it would find its way into the hands of those who lead health care organizations, those who work with and teach health care providers, to patients and families, and to members of the general public. Our hopes have been realized, and we have been encouraged to hear reports about how the book has led to innovative programs, changed institutional cultures, and touched people's lives.

For example, here's a sampling of what we have learned about how the book is being used and the impact it has had:

Catherine Aquino-Russell, a professor and program director on the Faculty of Nursing at the University of New Brunswick, Moncton Campus, uses *Privileged Presence* as a core text in her fourth-year course, Integrated Nursing Care. She reports that the response to the book is always enthusiastic and that a number of her students have told her that *Privileged Presence* is the first book they had read, cover to cover, in their whole university careers! They claim they "couldn't put it down." Additional student comments include the following:

"Each story reminded me of the importance of family, of small acts of caring, common sense, listening, responsibility, and meeting patients where they are as people."

"I have a renewed passion to learn everyone's story that makes them who they are."

"The stories have made me think of my own practice and they motivate me to make the extra effort to be caring and friendly, to listen, to have my eyes open to see the people in the hospital beds rather than simply doing the tasks needed and not acknowledging them as people."

"I feel I will be a better nurse because of *Privileged Presence*."

Dr. David Abelson, senior executive vice president of Health Partners and chief executive officer of Park Nicollet Health Services in Minneapolis, Minnesota, routinely opens meetings he chairs with a story from *Privileged Presence*.

Victoria Bayless, chief executive officer, and Sherry Perkins, chief operating officer/chief nursing officer of Anne Arundel Medical Center in Annapolis, Maryland, gave 150 copies of *Privileged Presence* to participants in a major planning retreat in 2010 to advance the practice of patient- and family-centered care. In 2014, this hospital earned the highest patient experience scores in the state of Maryland.

Dr. Linda Hofler, senior vice president/nurse executive, Vidant Medical Center, Vidant Health, Greenville, North Carolina, read *Privileged Presence* and immediately pondered "what it could be like to give voice to the stories that nurses and health care professionals that I work with hold in their hearts. The experiences of the providers stay with them for their entire career and shape who they become as a professional and a person. *Privileged Presence* inspired us to find our stories and give them value and meaning in shaping our patient- and family-centered culture."

Kathy Dutton, senior administrator of the Office of Patient-Family Experience at Vidant Medical Center, says, "We have learned to use stories strategically to enhance quality, safety, and experiences in care. Stories are shared at board meetings, manager and staff meetings, huddles, in hospital communications, and on the system's website. Thousands of our team hear stories every year at new employee, volunteer, and physician orientations, as well as at professional conferences. We published a collection of stories from nurses in 2011 entitled *Connections*, and we share a keepsake copy with every new nurse at our hospital."

Amy Jones, also with the Office of Patient-Family Experience at Vidant Health, adds "With heightened pressures to deliver on outcomes in the current health care environment, it could be easy to lose sight of the human connections and relationships occurring in hospitals, clinics, and community health settings each and every day. Stories keep us focused on the fact that each outcome is not a number but a person."

Linda Larin, chief administrative officer of the University of Michigan Cardiovascular Center, University of Michigan Health System (UMHS), in Ann Arbor, Michigan, says she first read *Privileged Presence* on a train and "read it all in one sitting with Kleenex in hand. It riveted my determination as a health care administrator and leader to try to improve the patient care experience. I came back to my institution and immediately purchased twenty-five books and gave them out to key leaders who could join me in "changing the world" of health care delivery at UMHS. This effort created sparks of enthusiasm and passion for patient- and family-centered care across the system." Linda also took on a personal challenge to bring UMHS patient stories to life to help spread the word and continue to inspire change. She succeeded with the 2014 publication of her book *Inspired to Change: Improving Patient Care One Story at a Time.*

What's New in the Second Edition?

All the original stories are still included in this second edition but two of them have been significantly revised. The story, which was titled "Lingering Effects" in the first edition, is now titled "When Loss Is Suppressed or Acknowledged." The original story captured a mother's experience of giving birth to a baby she knew was already dead. The new version conveys more about this experience. It now also includes a description of this same woman's daughter, decades later, going through a similar experience of birthing a baby she knew had died. This part of the story describes a dramatically different experience because the loss was honored and appropriate support was given. Juliette Schlucter's original story, "Creating a Culture," has been expanded and updated.

The original stories have been joined by nine new stories. The themes of the new stories range from the pain of restrictive visiting policies and the importance of listening to residents in a nursing home to interprofessional practice in action with a security department and views from leaders who have experienced care themselves.

The section titled "Building the Momentum for Change" has been fully updated in terms of organizations devoted to improving care and expanded in terms of useful tools for promoting change. Last but not least, the Selected Bibliography has been updated and reorganized.

What's Happening in the Field of Patient- and Family-Centered Care?

In recent years, a number of terms are being used, almost interchangeably, among those who are seeking to improve care. Such terms include *patient- and family-centered care, person-centered care, patient engagement,* and *the patient experience.* Although these concepts are closely interrelated, this book consistently uses the term *patient- and family-centered care* as the one term that most comprehensively and consistently refers to core values of an organization that guide planning, delivery, and evaluation of health care. Grounded in mutually beneficial partnerships among patients, families, and health care providers, these core concepts are respect and dignity, information sharing, participation, and collaboration.

The term *person-centered care* is often used to convey that not only are patients and families important, but staff is also important. Although it is true that everyone is important in mutually beneficial partnerships, it is even truer that health care institutions exist to care for patients and families and it is the role of staff to honor that purpose. The term *patient engagement* leaves out family and, at its simplest, infers that someone must engage the patient. This means that the relationship has a different fulcrum point than one that is a full collaborative partnership. And the term *patient experience* is simply descriptive of the result of the sum of all interactions shaped by an organization's culture that influence patient and family perceptions of care across the continuum of care. The term does not reflect standards or values and it is possible for a patient experience to be horrible.

Over the last decade, more and more individuals and organizations have realized the importance of creating a culture of patient- and family-centered care. In June, 2012, while speaking at the Fifth International Conference on Patient- and Family-Centered Care: Partnerships for Quality and Safety in Washington, D.C., Dr. Don Berwick said, "The most direct route to the Triple Aim is via patient- and family-centered care in its fullest form." It is increasingly understood that respectful and collaborative partnerships with patients, families, and health care providers lead to improving the experience of care, improving the health of populations, and reducing the costs of care.

Changing the culture of health organizations from being staff-centered to patient- and family-centered takes leadership and commitment over time. As Pat Sodomka, a senior health executive, taught us, "Leaders are responsible for the values of their organization. They are the guardians of the ideals of patient care." Leaders need to say that the signs labeling families as visitors and restricting family presence must come down; they need to convey that no evidence exists to support such restrictions, that staff have no right to keep loved ones apart; and that families are partners in care, not "visitors." Effective leaders model partnerships with patients and families and value and support the work and dedication of staff. These leaders also set standards for behaviors and attitudes and establish the systems of accountability. Leaders of high-performing health care organizations share stories to encourage and celebrate transformational change.

Stories play a role in creating a culture of collaboration and partnerships for quality and safety. Stories serve as doorways to discover and deeply appreciate our common humanity. We need to understand the stories of the patients and families we serve; we need to know the stories of our co-workers; and we need to remember that we have our own stories that we always carry with us. When we genuinely listen to someone's story or when we share our stories about our experiences, touching on both our joys and our sorrows, we are significantly changed. We hope the stories in this book will touch you, motivate you, and inspire you . . . and change you in the best ways possible.

Introduction

What Is Privileged Presence?

Why This Book?

What Matters in Health Care?

Why Stories?

Why These Stories?

Who Is This Book For?

What Is Privileged Presence?

Privileged Presence. One title, two words, three meanings.

Health care experiences are moments of "privileged presence." When people are dealing with illness or injury, their own or a loved one's, all their senses are intensified. Health care experiences are defining moments in people's lives, full of poignancy and power, and are remembered for years, often in vivid detail.

Health care professionals are *privileged* to be present with patients and families during these periods of heightened stress, which are characterized by courage, fear, uncertainty, and vulnerability.

When personal connections are made, then patients and families are also *privileged* to be in the presence of health care professionals, with their training, caring, and compassion.

And, last but not least, we have been *privileged* to be in the presence of those who were willing to open their hearts and share their personal stories for this collection.

Privileged Presence: Personal Stories of Connections in Health Care is a collection of more than sixty true stories about a wide range of health care experiences. At their core, the stories are all about people connecting with people or people missing the opportunity to connect.

The stories reflect different perspectives (patients, families, health care professionals) and a variety of health care situations and settings, from a seemingly ordinary and routine visit to a doctor's office to a highly charged and complex stay in intensive care. Some stories in this collection will disturb you; others will warm your heart.

You will see how the kindness of emergency personnel lifted a mother's spirits in a time of crisis; how a dismissive and arrogant professional undermined the confidence of an already vulnerable family; how a husband turned his sense of helplessness into a beautiful, caring way of providing support; how a parent struggled to make sense of her son's world of mental illness; how the many kindnesses experienced by a dying man motivated him to establish an organization to promote compassionate care; how two young parents were supported through the death of their firstborn child and the birth of their second; how a hospital administrator dealt with the tragedy of medical error; and how an elderly patient was "released" by her doctor for asking questions.

Why This Book?

The idea behind this book is simple and has been brewing for some time. We have shared more than four decades of friendship and professional collaboration. In our different roles as teachers, nurses, trustees, health care advisors, and even simulated patients, we have seen phenomenal extremes in how health care professionals treat patients and families, and the degree to which patients and families are able to express their views, be heard, and be invited into a partnership of care.

In addition to our professional work, we have also had babies, raised children, cared for aging parents, supported friends, and cried openly in the face of tragedy and death. Our personal experiences on the receiving end of health care, directly and with family members and friends, have underscored our belief that the delivery of health care needs to be more patient- and family-centered.

We have traveled unique paths in our two countries but have both worked locally, nationally, and internationally for changes in health care. We have spoken to large audiences, consulted in boardrooms, brought together people with conflicting views to build consensus, written articles, and produced documentary films.

Over the years, we have shared many stories about health care with each other. We have often mused, "If only everyone could hear these stories! Surely, then, people would see how important it is to connect fully with each individual patient, not just their illness." We have asked ourselves questions such as "How can families become empowered and understand that they have a right to ask questions?" or "Why are some health care professionals compassionate while others appear to be indifferent?"

At the same time, people were often asking us questions such as "Where can I get a book that describes what I'm going through? Where can I read about the health care experiences of others? Where can I learn from those who have shown the courage to bring about change?"

These questions of our friends and colleagues built on our own questions, and we finally asked ourselves, "Could a book of personal health care stories show the world what we have learned and care so much about? Could such a book be of value?" Our answer was to put together this collection.

One way to think of *Privileged Presence* is as a support group in a book. People want to know about others who have been there, who have gone down the same path, and who have some understanding about the experience.

The stories in *Privileged Presence* share the wisdom of personal experiences so that all readers can gain new insights. Some stories will provide the comfort of familiarity; some will inspire the confidence for patients to become actively engaged in their own health care; some will speak to the compassion of clinicians; some will evoke the courage and determination to make a change in a hospital practice or policy; and some will simply and quietly support intuition and instincts.

Although each story in *Privileged Presence* is different, they all echo the importance of honoring the uniqueness of patients and families and acknowledging their concerns, worries, and values. The collection as a whole offers powerful messages about the essential ingredients of "good" health care: respect; compassion; collaboration; open and honest communication; family support and involvement; and flexibility and responsiveness to individuals and their needs.

What Matters in Health Care?

Over the more than forty years we have known each other and worked together, we have become increasingly convinced that the common denominator in what makes a difference in health care is always people and how they communicate with and show respect for one another. We also believe:

- Patients and families have expertise, knowledge, and intuitive understanding about themselves.

- Health and illness affect not only individuals but also families, however an individual's *family* is defined.

- The patient is the most active participant in the healing process.

- Patients are more than a disease or injury.

- Honest communication and collaboration benefit everyone in health care partnerships.

- Health care is rooted, first and foremost, in human relationships. Medical technology and technical expertise are only tools within those relationships.

David Leach, MD, executive director of the Accreditation Council for Graduate Medical Education, when presenting an award related to fostering relationship-centered care, said that "all cooperative arts depend on relationship, and the number one problem in medicine today is finding a way to create the space where relationships can happen."

Clinical decision making must be rooted in human relationships. Medical equipment and clinical interventions, with all their advances to support diagnosis and treatment, should never replace or get in the way of genuinely listening to patients and families. Because medicine is an art as well as a science, relying only on medical science ignores the art of making human connections.

The desire for better connections in health care is neither frivolous nor inconsequential. There is a growing body of literature that reports improved outcomes for patients and families who are more informed, who participate actively in decisions about their health care, and who have practical and emotional support.

Many leaders in health care are reaching out to patients and families and inviting them to tell their stories and participate in everything from facility design planning to policy making. These connections and partnerships with patients and families are not just benefiting clinical encounters but are also enhancing the quality of care, ensuring patient safety, and improving patient satisfaction.

Why Stories?

We are an oral culture. We naturally tell stories to one another. Stories are a way of sharing our lives. When we tell stories, we find out what makes us unique and what makes us similar, what connects us and what builds bridges away from a world of pain and isolation. We feel a special sense of privilege when someone shares a particularly heartfelt story with us.

Talk to anyone who has just been diagnosed with an illness, or a spouse who spent the night in the emergency room waiting for news, or a mother whose son who is learning to cope with diabetes, and you will instantly hear a story. They will describe encounters and anecdotes and how the people who cared for them and their loved ones made a difference in their lives, both good and bad.

Sometimes the recounting of an event can be cathartic. For example, the mother in the story "I Needed a Guide" told us that the telling of her story helped her see that she had actually "done some things right" in the immediate aftermath of this tragic event and helped her replace her feelings of guilt with a sense of competence.

Sometimes telling your story is a doorway to someone else's story. For example, the mother in "I Want My Children with Me" told us that she was able to share her story with her younger daughter. This created the catalyst for surfacing her daughter's recollections of a day that she'd kept to herself for a long time.

Sometimes stories are powerful tools for change. For example, when the wife in "Flying Blind in a Frightening World" ultimately told her story to her husband's physician, the doctor began to change how he relates to his other patients.

And sometimes stories are powerful tools for learning. For example, the administrator in "Learning from Tragedy" told us that the most significant changes made in his hospital have come from involving, listening to, and learning from patients and families.

Rachel Naomi Remen, author of *Kitchen Table Wisdom*, has said that "Facts bring us to knowledge, but stories lead to wisdom." Stories often bring us closer to our own buried wisdom and remind us of our courage. Telling stories and hearing stories reassure us that we are not alone, that we are part of a richly textured human tapestry of experience, that we are in wonderful company.

Stories can be powerful medicine. Sharing experiences and feelings through stories helps us make sense of our lives and process trauma and loss. In gathering stories for this collection, in interview after interview, people would say, "Every time I tell my story, I feel a bit better." Hearts opened. Suffering diminished.

Why These Stories?

The personal stories we've gathered in this collection are both inspirational and instructive. Some are simply heartwarming and show how connections in health care can be positive. Some offer clinicians new insights about the experience of care. Others give readers pictures of courage and role models for having the confidence to speak up and to demand to be included in decisions about their health care. Still others stimulate reactions of outrage, serving as illustrations of what needs to change in health care practices.

Readers will meet a nurse who delights in seeing her staff bring a husband and wife together; a father who wants health care professionals to remember all that his son could once do; a doctor who believes in the power of a hug; a young woman left alone in labor; a medical student who feels compelled to put his values in storage; and a woman with bowel cancer who has nothing but praise for those who cared for her.

Virtually everyone has at least one health care story. People were more than willing to share their stories, to applaud the importance of compassion, and to showcase the harm of insensitivity. All the stories in *Privileged Presence* are true, but many names have been changed to protect privacy.

How did we choose the stories? We looked for experiences that were simple but powerful, diverse but resonating with a ring of the familiar. The stories chosen for this book were selected as ones that illustrate a range of experiences.

Many stories are so complex that they demonstrate both positive and negative aspects of care. Hopefully all will serve as inspiration for either what needs to be changed or what is possible.

The perspective presented in each story is that of the storyteller. In any given situation, there are always many different points of view; these personal narratives offer the storyteller's reality.

The stories are presented simply; they are plain, straightforward storytelling. The objective is to show rather than tell, to describe rather than preach. It is our hope that this unique and powerful collection of stories will touch readers in a variety of ways. Gentle wisdom is the objective.

Who Is This Book For?

Increasingly, the general public is expressing concern about the impersonality and complexity of health care. Patients and families want health care professionals to connect with them on a human and personal level and to be emotionally supportive.

Patients and families also comment that caregivers often don't provide either enough information or information they can understand; they want information so that they can make appropriate decisions about their health care. Additionally, people feel that the health care system is a nightmare to navigate and to understand; they feel they must have someone with them to protect and advocate for them.

Patients and families, as well as health care administrators, clinicians, educators, and policy makers, all want to know what they can do to bring about change. We hope this book will provide some answers.

This collection of health care stories shows what works and what does not, what people want and what they do not, and what adds to or takes away from people's sense of confidence and well-being in the context of health care experiences.

We hope this book will make a difference to individuals and families and how they see their roles in health care. We also hope it will touch the hearts and minds of the professionals who work in health care settings and help them see that when you become a health care professional, the responsibilities and opportunities to touch people's lives are extraordinary.

This book is for anyone and everyone who cares about the human condition and can relate to the world of health care. The stories are as equally relevant to all those who have had a health care experience as they are to those who want to see changes in the health care system.

The stories can be read in private and reflected upon alone, or they can be the focal points for group discussions, raising such questions as "What would I/you have done?"; "What was done well?"; "What needs to be different?"; "How does this story relate to what we are doing in our clinics and hospitals and what can we learn from it?"

Introduction

We believe that you will be touched by the truth and wisdom contained in these pages. We cannot presume to know what meanings readers will take from these stories or how the book as a whole will affect their lives. What we do know is that these stories have inspired us.

~

As Unique as Snowflakes: Responding to Individuals

"I was surprised that people with the same disease had such very different stories."
—*Rachel Naomi Remen*

"People in their most vulnerable states still just want to be people."
—*Suzy Crocker*

"People will forget what you said, people will forget what you did, but people will never forget how you made them feel."
—*Maya Angelou*

~

Illness and injury can create feelings of enormous vulnerability. In these circumstances, patients and family members long for someone to help them make sense of their upside-down world and relate to them, one on one, person to person, seeing them for all they are . . . not just an illness or injury.

Health care professionals may have seen thousands of broken arms, respiratory infections, gastrointestinal problems, strokes . . . but for each person who walks into a doctor's office, a health care clinic, or a hospital, what they are experiencing is unique to them. Their pain is personal, their fears are their very own, their ordered lives are now disoriented.

No two people, situations, stories are the same. Each individual wants to be seen, heard, acknowledged, understood, and recognized as a whole person, with a name and with a life. Such recognition creates the foundation for respect and dignity which, in turn, are the pillars for a caring connection.

I Am Not a Patella

Aunt Mary

Respect for Dignity

Friends in Low Places

Who Will Walk the Dog?

Unriddling the Riddle

The Walk of Honor

Security Equals Safety with Sensitivity

I Am Not a Patella

IT WAS A TUESDAY EVENING and a regular modern-dance class. I was sixteen. I did a big *fouetté* (pivot) with big momentum across the room, but my foot stuck on the special floor covering used for dancers while my body kept going. I heard a pop. My leg was at a funny angle, and one of the teachers straightened it, but my kneecap was still in the wrong place. The pain was excruciating.

The ambulance guys were nice, but I felt every pothole on the way to the hospital. I waited in emergency for a long time with ice on my leg but with nothing else to numb the pain. About six hours later, the verdict was in. My kneecap (called a *patella*) was on the side of my leg. Surgery would be needed to put it back in place, but there was too much swelling to operate right away. Surgery was scheduled for Thursday morning. In the meantime, my leg was wrapped in a padded splint. The hospital staff thought I'd be more comfortable waiting at home.

My mum and I wondered how I'd even get into the car, let alone into the house and up the stairs at home. But home we went at 3 a.m., via an all-night drugstore for crutches. It was freezing cold and snowing outside. When we pulled up to my house, we first talked our way through how this would work. I couldn't lower my leg without experiencing shards of pain in my leg, and so while I would try to use the new crutches, my mum would hold my injured leg up at a right angle to my body. With ice on the pathway, it was going to be tricky. A poor, unsuspecting newspaper delivery man ended up helping us navigate from the car to the front door.

When Thursday came, I was excited about the surgery because I wanted to have my knee put back the way it should be. Of course, I don't remember too much after surgery because I was groggy, but

I do know it was exciting to get a TV and embarrassing to use the bedpan. And I knew my mum was staying in my room overnight. Apparently, the nurses told her that was okay, but there were no cots, so she created a sleeping surface by lining up two footstools and a chair and brought a sleeping bag and pillow from home. (Ironically, on the last morning, after three nights, a new nurse came in when my mum was taking her "bed" apart and said, "Goodness! You could have had a cot, you know!" Go figure!)

The next morning, a doctor I'd never met before came into my room with a bunch of other people and said to his group, "So, this is the patella." I tried to respond with, "Yeah, I'm Suzy," but he didn't respond to me. Did he think I wasn't there? He never told me who he was and never spoke to me by name. He just spewed out medical jargon to the doctors with him. I felt like a science experiment.

Didn't he know I was desperate for more information about what had happened and what would happen to my body? He was supposed to be looking after me, but I did not feel comfortable with him. How can you feel comfortable with someone who doesn't look you in the eye, shake your hand, call you by name, and tell you who they are?

Next, a physical therapist came in. All orders and no sympathy. She told me to get out of bed. This was the first time in four days that I had lowered my leg below 90 degrees. I've always believed that if something is super painful, then it probably isn't good for you. My leg hurt a lot and I was scared. She offered no alternatives as to what I could do. She just left.

Fortunately, I got a different therapist the next day who was nice. She asked how my leg felt and if I was nervous. She was so encouraging and told me to just take my time. She actually showed me what she wanted me to do and how to safely approach the movements. I felt comfortable with her. She seemed to understand that, at the end of the day, it's about two people in a room trying to solve the same problem together.

The nurses were pretty cool. They showed me some little tricks to make it easier to move my leg, and one of them, even though I was going to be discharged later in the day, washed my hair. I can't tell you how good that felt! People in their most vulnerable states still just want to be people.

.....

Suzy recovered fully and went on to dance again.

Aunt Mary

My Aunt Mary was a life-long spinster who always lived independently. Even growing up, I knew she was a force to be reckoned with. Aunt Mary was right even when she was wrong. I loved her, I respected her, and I was a little bit afraid of her. And so when she called me to say, "I want to go to the hospital tomorrow," I paid attention. I don't know why I bothered suggesting a closer hospital because Aunt Mary was set on the hospital she wanted. She was also specific about "tomorrow" because she was working that day, looking after a ninety-year-old woman.

When I picked her up, I could see that Aunt Mary was jaundiced. After evaluation in the emergency department, it was clear she wouldn't be going home. This would be Aunt Mary's first time in the hospital. Because she had no frame of reference for that world, she had some unusual conversations.

For example, one day she told me, "This place is so stupid. Some doctor was saying I should have a face-lift. I told him I didn't want one and to leave." I was eventually able to figure out that "some doctor" had been a hematologist who had been suggesting that Aunt Mary have some "platelets." Somehow, all she heard was "face-lift."

On another occasion, a doctor was trying to find out what Aunt Mary would like in terms of "do not resuscitate" orders. The doctor must not have been clear enough for her to conclude that he was talking about her. She reported, "This doctor was telling me all these awful stories about what they have to do to people sometimes. It all seemed gloomy, and so I asked him if he had a happy family. He said 'yes,' so I told him he should go home and spend some time with them."

And then one day, a social worker called me to tell me, "Your aunt is very frustrating. She won't have any care." They hit a road-block, and instead of trying to negotiate the barrier with her, they called me instead. I told them that if they were talking to me, they obviously hadn't talked to Aunt Mary. I couldn't and wouldn't speak for Aunt Mary. Rather, I suggested that, if they asked her some questions, they might discover Aunt Mary rarely had an unclear thought, felt she'd had an exceptional eighty-seven years of life, and wasn't interested in any of the hospital's invasive procedures.

Aunt Mary never wanted to be in the hospital, but we prom-ised her she would never be alone. She was always surrounded by Irish music and family and friends. Even when Aunt Mary slipped into a coma, there were still people with her.

Initially, the nurses had been resistant about our being there all the time, citing some rule. As soon as I pushed a bit, though, the nurses caved in and brought chairs for us. The staff talked about how atypical it was to have people there all the time, but they could see how comfortable Aunt Mary was. I felt so badly for all the other patients who spent their nights alone with the dark.

Respect for Dignity

MY MOTHER-IN-LAW, EDITH, IS EIGHTY-NINE and suffers from a lot of pain from arthritis. Fortunately, Edith found a family practitioner who truly honors her wishes and requests.

When Edith goes for her regular physical, she doesn't go in and immediately get undressed. The visit starts with a chat. Her doctor says, "I need to talk to you first to figure out what we might want to do today." He always talks at eye level with her.

When the issue of an annual mammogram came up recently, the doctor reminded Edith of this diagnostic procedure. She said, "I've lived too long as it is. I certainly don't want any more mammograms." He replied, "I understand. It is my duty to tell you about it, but I respect your choice not to do it."

~

Edith experienced the same respect for her dignity when she went to our small community hospital for surgery on her wrist for carpal tunnel syndrome. When she arrived, the nurses noticed that Edith was quite crippled by arthritis. They said she could stay seated in her wheelchair and asked her only to take off her blouse and put on a hospital gown, which rested on the rest of her street clothes. (She didn't even have to take off her bra.)

The nurses took her right into the operating room in her wheelchair and brought her back out again in the same chair after surgery. She never had to get out of her street clothes! Noticing the puzzled look on my face, the nurses said, "Oh, we've checked the literature. There's nothing to worry about with street clothes for this small surgical procedure."

Friends in Low Places

MY FIRST ENCOUNTER WITH PETER was prompted by a phone call on Thanksgiving Day 1994. My sister, brother-in-law, and I were just about to go for an early morning walk when a patient called me on my cell phone to tell me that there was "a guy in bad shape in the old dry-cleaning building" and asked if I would please go and help him.

At this point in time, I had been working as a nurse practitioner at the clinic of a local shelter on Cape Cod for about a year. I was the first full-time provider and the first to work during the day. Staffing up to that time had consisted of volunteer physicians and nurses two evenings per week. Daytime hours were for outreach and continuity of care. I spent my first year going out on the streets and seeking out places where the homeless congregated. This became the cornerstone of my practice, and that Thanksgiving Day phone call was testimony to the fact that my approach was working.

I proposed to my sister and brother-in-law that we walk to the dry-cleaning building. They conceded but wondered why we needed to do this on a holiday. "Thanksgiving Day?" I replied, "What better day to help out someone less fortunate!"

Thirty minutes later we were looking into the open door of the old dry-cleaning building. Mattresses, bedding, several sleeping bags, blankets, and empty liquor bottles were strewn about. The place was dark and smelled of urine and stale beer. I stepped in and began looking around. My relatives watched anxiously at the doorway.

At first it seemed that the building was empty, but then I heard someone moaning. I moved closer to the sound, and there, under a pile of blankets, was a man who looked to be in his seventies with long white hair and a full beard. "Hello," I said. He replied,

"Who are you?" I told him my name and where I worked. He was not pleased and cursed as he attempted to stand. He was highly intoxicated and had obviously not bathed, changed his clothes, or shaved in a very long time.

It turned out that Peter was fifty-nine years old and had been living on the streets for several years. This initial encounter was the beginning of several years of engagement, trust building, and eventual medical management of several medical issues related to Peter's acute and chronic alcohol and substance abuse. These complications included bilateral hearing loss; depression; post-traumatic stress disorder (PTSD); personality disorder; chronic alcoholic hepatitis; peripheral neuropathy; exposure resulting in frostbite, gangrene, and amputation of his right big toe, as well as other toe debridement; multiple bouts of pneumonia; pancreatitis; skin cancer; peptic ulcer disease; multiple trauma related to falls and assaults, with resultant degenerative lumbar-sacral disc disease and lumbar osteoarthritic changes; and foot drop.

Peter's gait was unsteady, and he soon fell back to the ground. He went to the hospital that day against his will. From that encounter on, however, we began a relationship as patient and provider that eventually turned into friendship. Our relationship was often difficult because Peter had many issues regarding trust due to a very abusive childhood. But persistence and consistency in my work with him helped him to learn to trust me.

In reality, we had a lot in common. We both grew up in Boston, we both were Irish Catholic, and we both had had an alcoholic parent. The difference between us was "There but for the grace of God. . . ."

Giving Peter unconditional love allowed him to grow as a person. Peter had a great smile, a quick wit, and a kind heart when given the chance to express his humanity. Sober, he was able to demonstrate compassion toward others and would often bring in snacks and little gifts to the clinic staff.

Peter struggled with his addiction and at one point achieved eighteen months of sobriety while living in a halfway house. The real success came in January 2000, however. After being arrested while intoxicated, Peter decided to go into treatment one more time, and he never drank again.

In 2001, Peter decided to move to Pennsylvania. A friend who was a minister had agreed to help him find housing. Peter would call me every few months or so. In September 2005, he called to tell me he had a new apartment. He was happy, still sober, and connected with a church. He inquired about my family and gave me his new phone number, promising to stay in touch.

In early November 2005, I received a call from the shelter stating that a Peter K. had been found dead in his apartment in Pennsylvania. The coroner's office wanted to know if we knew of any next of kin. Review of his medical records from the local hospital revealed that Peter had listed me as his next of kin. I am in the process of having him cremated, and his ashes will be shipped to me. Once I am in possession of his remains, I plan to have a service for him.

Many of his homeless brothers and sisters will join me, as we have so often done in the past, to pray for Peter, and we will scatter his ashes in the sea. Although I feel sad for the life that might have been, I am confident that Peter did find hope and joy in the end.

·····

The nurse practitioner in this story has worked for twelve years to bring healing to the homeless, the underserved, and those who have been left behind. Her outreach efforts have taken her on to the streets, inside derelict buildings, and into the woods. She says, "I have friends in very low places."

Over a number of years, her efforts expanded from an intermittent, weekly, one-woman nursing service to a full-time multiservice medical health clinic with twenty employees. This energetic and tireless woman explains that she eventually became burned out from dealing with bureaucracy and administrative tasks and so stepped down as clinical director.

"I need to be able to talk to people. Everyone has a story, and I love to listen and help people figure things out. I never suffer from 'compassion fatigue' as long as I can work directly with those in need."

She believes that simple acts of healing can occur with each concerned question, caring visit, and reassuring touch. She bemoans the fact that many nurses never get to give baths or backrubs anymore. "That's when you hear what's really on people's minds and in their hearts."

Who Will Walk the Dog?

ODD THINGS SOMETIMES CAME ACROSS MY DESK when I was working as the hospital's legal counsel in risk management. One of my favorites was the request about a dog.

The charge nurse from the general medicine unit came to see me to find out if there was any legal reason why a patient couldn't have her dog stay in the hospital with her. My "lawyer" response was, "Probably not, so long as we get the proper release forms signed," but because I had been a nurse before becoming a lawyer, I was curious about the clinical circumstances.

It was quite simple. A woman who used a wheelchair had been admitted. She wanted to have her "helper" dog with her.

As nurses we often refer to what we call "the evil-twin response"—you know, the response you might want to give but you know is wrong—and you always hope that when you open your mouth, the "good twin" will be speaking. In this case, the "evil-twin response" would have been, "You don't need the dog. We're doing everything for you." It was, however, the "good twin" who showed up in my office that day.

The "good twin" knew that you have to take patients as you find them. In this case, the woman had no family or friends. Her dog was everything to her and maybe the only living being who loved her.

To make a long story short, the dog was admitted. The patient was set up in a private room, and the charge nurse hired a dog walker out of the unit's budget.

Unriddling the Riddle

OUR FIRSTBORN SON WAS BORN FIFTEEN YEARS AGO with Down's syndrome. If we were upset about this, it was for less than forty-five seconds. We both very quickly realized that this was an opportunity and a blessing for us. Our early years with our son proved us right. I remember saying, "I can deal with Down's syndrome, but I don't know how the parents of a child with autism cope." Little did I know I would have the chance to find out.

Our son had extensive language and played on the same soccer team as his younger brother. In developmental language, his "global functioning" was 85 percent. Around his ninth birthday, though, we entered a nightmarish world. He started behaving strangely. In a matter of three or four months, he lost all language, stopped eating or dressing himself, and no longer prompted for going to the bathroom. His global functioning deteriorated to 10 to 15 percent.

We had no idea what was going on. Was this a psychological problem? Was it psychiatric in origin? Was it a developmental phenomenon? We turned everywhere for ideas and answers.

We had just moved to a new city. This meant that our son's doctors had not known him before, but we had video footage of him before his behavior changed so dramatically. In it, our son was talking and laughing and interacting. We used this video to impress on specialists that there was a once-happy boy inside this nonresponsive person.

A year after our son's functional slide backward, when he was ten, he had surgery to address stomach problems he'd been having for some time. After this surgery, he dramatically improved and experienced a steep rise out of his doldrums. He returned to about 75 percent functioning in six weeks. Then, as quickly as he had returned, he went back down into his hole again. For the past five years, his highest functioning has been 25 percent.

We decided to move back home, to the city and the specialists who had worked with our son before his functioning deteriorated. We wanted to be close to people who would be as driven as we were to try to make him better. When you have known a child who has been healthy and functioning and who then mysteriously declines, it provides powerful motivation to work to get this child back.

It's a lesson in human nature to understand that medical professionals are far more tenacious and thoughtful when they have an emotional connection to the potential improvements they can bring about. Our son's principal specialist was completely aligned with us emotionally, even when she was hitting brick walls. Like us, she wouldn't give up.

Some specialists have given up, which is frustrating. It's as though they've run through their standard treatments and, if nothing has worked, they want to move on to another person. Where's their curiosity? Why don't they want to try to turn over new stones? I believe our son is a riddle that needs to be unriddled.

I worry that we are missing the boat entirely. I can't help but believe that the secret to this riddle lies somewhere in the body-mind connection, in the gut-brain connection. We have researched as much as we can through the Internet and are now trying to secure a referral to a specialist in Massachusetts.

We are in the middle of this battle right now. It forms the context of our lives. We are battle weary. Just talking about it is a challenge.

I lie beside my son and listen to his stomach making noises like the Fourth of July. One of the hardest things for me is thinking that our son has been in chronic, constant, and terrible pain for years. I saw it on his face this morning.

We have two other sons. They love their older brother dearly and have learned that "we are all beautiful in our own ways." They play with their brother, cuddle with him, and rub his back and his belly. When they pray at night, they pray for their brother and to become professional hockey players. They tell God that if He has to make a choice, they want Him to make their brother better.

What would I like to say to health care professionals if I had one hundred of them in a room?

- Make your best efforts to be present for your patients in every way. You can be buried by these things, but the more you are present in the moment rather than processing, the better the experience for the patient and family.

- Know that patients and families can sense whether you are fully engaged and listening.

- Listen carefully to what parents say about their children's symptoms. Parents have insights and know subtleties of their kids that can help doctors figure out what to do.

Is our son autistic? I don't know, in part because he seems more socially engaged than is typical for autistic children. We're told that he has a "chronic disintegrative disorder."

The most important thing right now is to think outside the box and to let go of ordinary expectations. It is said that you can't get clarity unless you embrace the confusion. I worry that the last five or six years in this state have deeply patterned our son. I pray that we can unriddle this riddle before he becomes stuck.

The Walk of Honor

OUR NINETY-SIX-BED NURSING HOME is divided into six sixteen-bed "households," and each household holds weekly "learning circles." Someone picks a topic and everyone in the circle can comment. There's no interrupting until everyone has a chance to speak.

On this particular day, I don't even know if dealing with dying was the topic of the day. I just know that one of our residents spoke up saying, "When someone dies here, why do you sneak them out the back door? Why do you wait until we're not looking?" Someone else chimed in, "The people who die here are my friends. I'd like to say 'good-bye.' " Another voice reasoned, "Do you think we don't know we're going to die? We're old. Of course, we're going to die!" And then a quiet voice questioned, "Are you going to do that to me?"

Years before this day, when we were designing a remodel of our facility, we paused and asked ourselves, "Would we want to live here?" Our answer had been a resounding, "No." And so we went back to the drawing board and invited the current residents and families as well as the community to tell us what they would want in a nursing home. And they told us: they wanted four-season porches; they wanted to sleep until they naturally woke up; they wanted to eat when they wanted; they wanted visitors of all ages, including pets; they wanted a cup of coffee when they felt like it; they wanted to take their medications and baths when they were used to doing so at home.

We built what they asked for, knowing that we needed to change more than the building. We also needed to change the model of care. People had told us that they wanted to oust the rigidity of schedules and roles. We cross-trained staff so each direct care employee was responsible for nursing, housekeeping, laundry, dietary needs, and activities and could meet the immediate needs of what individual residents needed.

The results have been astounding. The majority of residents gained weight; the number of folks suffering from falls plummeted; call lights were answered faster; the number of people needing assistance to eat meals is way down; and restraints have become a thing of the past. We were now not just focusing on the quality of care but also on the quality of life.

We were proud of our accomplishments. We had changed so much, but we hadn't changed what we did when someone dies. Appropriately, our residents told us what they wanted. First, there were to be no body bags. And then each household decided what they wanted to do. One household has chosen for everyone to put a flower on the deceased person's bed; another household has every resident write down their memories of the person, and the collection of memories is given to the family at the funeral; and in another household, the residents gather together in a circle around the person who died and share stories out loud.

Every household has a "Walk of Honor." The person who has died is covered with a "Dignity Quilt," the residents line the hallway, and their former friend is wheeled out the front door. The family members are as involved as they want to be—some want to wash the body; some want to drape their family member with the quilt; and some just want to help push the cart.

The impact of this single change, the "Walk of Honor," is enormous. It has changed our view of death from something one might be afraid of or want to hide to one of openness, comfort, and acceptance. One son commented, "Thanks so much for this. I've never been part of a more moving experience. Sadly, the last memory of my mum, years ago, was her being taken out of the room in a zippered bag."

· · · · ·

Chuck Hofius is the chief executive officer of Perham Health, an integrated continuum of health provision in rural west central Minnesota. Perham Health includes Perham Living, a ninety-six-bed nursing home, as well as a twenty-five-bed acute care hospital and a number of clinics. Chuck says that the practice of the "Walk of Honor" has now also been adopted by the acute care hospital.

Security Equals
Safety with Sensitivity

A SITUATION IN MY EARLY DAYS at the hospital touched me deeply. At the time, in our emergency department, the entrance was reserved strictly for emergency department patients, families, and visitors. No one else was allowed to use it; others were referred to other entrances. This particular night, a family had rushed to the hospital because they'd been notified that a family member was gravely ill in intensive care. They tried to enter through the emergency department entrance, but the security officer turned them away, directing them to an entrance they could access from the parking structure. Tragically, this family got lost, and by the time they found their way to intensive care, their family member had died. I felt this was wrong, and I knew we could do better. The opportunity to change presented itself.

In 2005, C. S. Mott Children's and Women's Hospital established a Patient- and Family-Centered Care (PFCC) Committee. Our security staff became educated about PFCC, and its principles became embedded in our own policies, protocols, and training. We learned what it means to treat people with respect and dignity, how to communicate clearly and listen intently, and how to determine what is important to patients and families. Along the way, we had to unlearn some of our language and judgments—we had to abandon terms like *drunks* and *crazy* and look behind people's behaviors and ask ourselves, "What does this person need right now?"

One of the early initiatives of our Patient- and Family-Centered Care Committee related to family presence and visitation. I believe security can make or break the case for 24/7 family presence and need to be involved. By supporting the good intentions and by identifying ways to deal with difficult situations, we contributed to the successful implementation of the 24/7 Family Presence and Visitation policy:

- We outlined ways to deal with visitor restrictions when "personal protection orders" exist or when patients and families make a choice to limit access.

- We were always available to assist when exceptions needed to be made.

- We developed "behavioral contracts" when necessary so that selected individuals would know what behaviors could lead to forfeiting their rights for 24/7 access.

- We provided assurance to the staff that they would be safe.

We also developed a new role of guest service specialist (GSS) for our women's and children's hospital. More than greeters or receptionists, our GSSes screen everyone who comes through our doors to ensure they have a legitimate reason to be there, issue them the appropriate badge, conduct infection-control screening, cross-reference their name against a visitor restriction list, and provide information and directions. GSSes are also positioned at the entrance to each patient floor where they perform the same functions. The security staff are part of the team on every unit.

Every officer goes through a day-long psychological screening process to ensure they meet our high standards for intelligence, critical thinking, communication skills, and the ability to inter-act with others appropriately. We practice simulations to help us learn to effectively deal with people with mental illness or autism or dementia. We develop skills to defuse situations and to prevent escalation.

Overall, our role is to greet people and help at entrances, help people with way finding, keep the physical plant and the staff secure, and resolve complaints. We provide special assistance (with a PFCC touch) for people who have to be physically managed such as patients who are detoxing, delusional, or demented. We are called for every code, for every arriving trauma situation, and we have both a behavior response team and an autism spectrum disorder (ASD) team.

The autism spectrum disorder (ASD) team grew out of the work of a multidisciplinary work group we established in 2009. We were being frequently asked to restrain children and adolescents, and we wanted better options. Parents of children with ASD were clearly the experts and, with their guidance, we were able to raise awareness about ASD for point-of-care staff and created a coping kit with useful items to help focus and calm patients.

Moments of extreme crisis occur every day, several times a day for individuals and families in hospitals. These moments are fraught with stress and danger. The potential for escalation to violence is always present; the need for comfort and calm is also always present. A security department that practices patient- and family-centered care and treats patients and families with compassion, empathy, dignity, and respect is the safest method for preventing and mitigating problems. From a security standpoint, it just makes sense. From a human standpoint, it is simply the right thing to do.

The following stories illustrate what patient- and family-centered care practiced by a security organization looks like. These stories represent the everyday, routine work of our security team, which does very special work on behalf of our patients and families.

The Gentle Giant of Psychiatric Emergency Services

An eight-year-old boy with severe autism was a patient in a seclusion room in the psychiatry emergency services department. He was waiting to be taken to an inpatient unit, but I was told he was very agitated and needed to be calmer before a transport could safely occur. I was on duty and was faced with the choice of either holding the boy down or restraining him until medication took effect. I didn't like either option, and so I decided to try to tire him out. I used to be an offensive lineman in college, so I held my hands in a boxing sparring position and allowed the boy to engage me until he became tired. It was the safest choice and resulted in a peaceful and uneventful trip to the inpatient unit.

Singing as a Security Tool

I witnessed something amazing today. A patient was hitting his back violently against a gurney that was set at an angle. Doctors feared he would hurt himself. Medication was given, but he continued to repeatedly throw his back against the gurney. The security officer held the gurney for a while to help protect the patient from getting hurt, but this security officer had had training about the needs of those with autism, and so he recognized this patient's autistic behaviors. He suggested that everyone sing to help the patient relax. A cell phone was turned to music and the officer sang. This helped calm the young man until the medication finally took effect, and he fell asleep.

Seek to Understand

At the end of a very difficult interaction with a patient's mother, the doctor, a surgeon, asked me what type of training I had received.

He said he had never seen someone able to calm a mother down once she had reached such a level of anger and dissatisfaction! I told him that we do get customer service training but patient- and family-centered care training was much more significant. I explained that customer service training taught me how to handle a complaint, but PFCC training actually taught me how to understand the complaint, how to understand the stress levels, and what it must have been like to feel the way she did when staff made negative comments. Without PFCC training, I would have handled it differently and would not have been so open to listening to the mother and trying to understand what she was feeling.

A Little Bit of Peace

I like to use my breaks during my twelve-hour shift to play the piano in the hospital's main lobby. A few months ago, while playing, I noticed a couple sitting in the lobby. The woman was quite distraught. She looked as if she had been crying, and I speculated they may have received some bad news. As I continued to play, the man approached me and asked if I knew how to play anything by Adele because his wife was a big fan. The man then explained their child was going to be taken off life support that day and that maybe a song would bring some peace to his wife at such a difficult time. Regrettably, I wasn't familiar with anything by Adele.

On my way back from break, however, I found some of Adele's music on YouTube and started to think about how I could play it on the piano.

When I returned to play the piano again, on my next break, I noticed the same couple was still there. I decided to try one of the Adele songs I had heard on YouTube. I began and looked over to the couple. The man was seated with his arm around his wife as she stared out at the courtyard. He looked back at me and gave me a "thumbs up." In that moment, I knew I had brought a little bit of peace to two people who were going through what might have been the most difficult day of their lives.

Why Security Officers Respond to Cardiac Arrests

I was dispatched to a code. When I arrived on the floor, a lot of people had gathered for the code, and the patient's mother was in the room with her daughter. The parents of the other patient in the room where the child had coded were standing in the hallway, visibly scared and upset. Not only could they not get to their child, but also, they had become friends with the girl and her family. I took them down to the waiting room and kept giving them updates. I was able to tell them their child was fine and sleeping through the code.

I was told that the patient was not doing well and that a social worker was needed. When the social worker arrived on the floor, I briefed her and walked her to the room.

Meanwhile, I was told that the child's father was on his way, and so I called the two after-hours' entrances and alerted the security officers there. I then chose to go directly to the entrance I thought he was most likely to come through.

Unfortunately, before he arrived, his twelve-year-old daughter lost her fight for her life. At least I was there to meet him and rush him to the floor to be with his family.

•••••

Perry Spencer joined the University of Michigan Hospitals and Health Centers (UMHHC) security and entrance services department in 1997 having previously served for twenty years in the United States Air Force Security Police. In 1999, he was named the department's manager of uniform operations.

Perry has incorporated patient- and family-centered care training as a staple of his security team's competencies, which has infused PFCC core principles into their daily operations. He says, "I believe our people are special, and it is reflected in their behavior and how they perform their jobs. I'm so very proud of our team and, although I know I am biased, I believe we have the best health care security force in the world!"

When Life Is Threatened: The Importance of Support

"Great opportunities to help others seldom come.
But small ones surround us every day."
—*Sally Koch*

"We cannot all do great things; but we can
do small things with great love."
—*Mother Teresa*

"A terminal illness affects the whole family,
and the entire family needs support."
—*Sue Uteck*

Support in health care situations comes in the same
ways it is offered in ordinary day-to-day life—
concerned questions, reassuring touches, sincere
listening, shared information, gentle truth, encouraging
words. Sometimes, people suffering from illness
or injury know how to ask for support, but others
can be intimidated by the system, overwhelmed by
their situation, or mired in a sense of unworthiness.
Especially for them, support must be offered.

Support matters. Who among us does not respond
to kindness, to concern, to love? When illness or
injury strikes, a literal or figurative hand to hold, a
shoulder to cry on, a functioning mind are needed.
Without support, people fare less well, recover
more slowly, and suffer the additional trauma
of being ignored, dismissed, or abandoned.

Death—Life

I sat in shock as the surgeon
Uttered the dreaded word
Cancer

He said other things—like "highly treatable"
All I could hear for the time was
Cancer

I sat there trying to take it in
Or block it out
Cancer

I imagined he was anxious to get it out
And me out of his office
Cancer

What now? Wander out of the hospital
Tears flowing unheeded
Cancer

The word echoes in my head
Over and over and over
Cancer

I feel the urge to stop strangers
And tell them
"I have Cancer"

When Life Is Threatened: The Importance of Support

I know my world will change
Never be exactly the same again
Cancer

What emotions are evoked by that word
Fear, sadness, grief, anger
All of the above

First overwhelming sadness
Then fear for my people
Then surrender

My guides gather round
To make themselves felt
And to comfort

I am filled with a sense
Of love and protection
Of knowing

A sense that this world is only temporary
That there is no death
Just going home

When my time comes—my guides will be there
Reaching out to embrace me
And welcome me home

June 2004

The sharing of this poem occurred in a coffee shop at the very beginning of the interview. Moments passed in silence, the reader slowly digesting how effectively the words have captured the shattering intensity of hearing the word *cancer*. The poem's author, a professional woman of sixty-three years, then said, "Every person who came into my life, from the point of this diagnosis on, was an angel."

Stella had had surgery to remove what she thought had been a persistent hemorrhoid that had been causing her extreme pain for two years. She was thrilled with the surgery because she could finally sit comfortably. This was her primary thought as she went to see her surgeon for a follow-up appointment.

He looked uncomfortable and said, "I have a surprise for you. This was cancer and I didn't get it all." He immediately added, "But it is 90 percent curable."

The poem captures the early moments and days . . . on to the angels.

> When I went through the double doors of the Cancer
> Care Clinic, I felt completely cared for in every way. I
> was welcomed, and my daughter was welcomed. I was
> given a journal to record details of my treatments. The
> journal also contained every possible phone number
> I might want as well as a twenty-four-hour number I
> could call for anything—anything at all.
>
> The radiation oncologist sat with me and my daugh-
> ter and answered every question I had. He spoke directly
> to me and also included her. He never looked at his
> watch. He covered everything—practical suggestions
> regarding what kind of underwear I would need and pre-
> scriptions for medications I might need. He even covered

really embarrassing things. It was as though he and the staff there had thought of everything for you because they didn't want you to have any unnecessary stress.

My biggest fear had been that I might have to deal with arrogant idiots and be vulnerable to them. The doctors and all the other staff were more than I could have hoped for—completely kind, personable, and interested in all of me.

I have nothing but praise for the Cancer Care Clinic. I never had to wait, and there was even a fast track for getting our blood taken at the blood lab. The clinic area was as attractive as it could be (given all the necessary special equipment), and there was also a place called the Sunshine Room. This looked like a living room, and there was always someone there to talk to you, to give a massage or reflexology treatment, to lend you a wig or scarf. This was a public clinic, but I felt like a valued customer at a fancy private clinic.

I am interested in alternative medicine, and when I asked about different options, the staff would say they didn't know about this or that but never were negative about my questions. When I brought in something a friend had recommended, the staff had a pharmacist look at it for me. He took the time to examine every ingredient to see if it would be compatible with what I was already taking.

I was really anxious about radiation. I thought it would be humiliating, thinking I'd have to have my legs somehow wrapped around my neck. The staff showed me that it would be much simpler and more dignified than I had thought. I had twenty-five treatments, and, on the day of the last treatment, I came out and all the technicians were lined up to hug me.

The clinic showed everyone so much kindness. They were completely committed to every aspect of the whole person. I felt totally looked after.

There were things I did for myself, too. For example, I filled my balcony with flowers. I did guided imagery and listened to tapes for relaxation and pain. I also listened to a forgiveness tape that I think has added ten years to my life. My family had a "Spoil Stella Day." And my own spiritual practice was important. My spirit guides offered me a lot of unconditional love and support, assuring me that I'd be okay either way. They told me that if I wanted to stay, I'd be fine, and if not, I'd be coming home to them.

Do I have any advice for others? I would say, be prepared to be patient, stay in the moment, and live one day at a time. That's all we ever have . . . just one day at a time. And it can be a good day or a bad day. We can decide.

· · · · ·

Stella still goes for checkups every three months. Stella and her husband, Paul, have recently bought a house that she feels is her way of saying "yes" to her future.

Flying Blind in a Frightening World

In the 1930s, a baseball player, New York Yankees' first baseman Lou Gehrig was diagnosed with amyotrophic lateral sclerosis, or ALS. This disease has come to be more commonly known as Lou Gehrig's disease. In the late 1990s, a former Canadian Football League player, my husband, was diagnosed with this same disease.

ALS is a terrifying disease. It usually begins in the lower body and rises, wasting muscles as it moves, until moving, swallowing, speaking, and eventually breathing become impossible. A person with ALS knows all this because the mind is unaffected.

What was the worst of it? My list is so long, but near the top would be the specialist. He may have had a lot of degrees, but he didn't know how to help us and he had the social skills of a newt! The higher in the medical food chain you go, the more mysterious doctors become. I discovered that just because they have lots of degrees doesn't mean they have any common sense.

In July 1996, my husband noticed that one of his hands had started shaking. Our family doctor didn't think this was anything to worry about at first. My husband, from his days playing professional football, had a number of crushed vertebrae in his neck, and it was assumed that the shaking was a residual effect of the damage to his neck. As the months passed, though, there were other troubling changes. I can still remember the day we had a huge fight about tying his tie. He had had to ask for help and didn't like how I was doing it—not a happy scene!

I remember going to the specialist with my husband in January 1997. He had had a number of tests for Parkinson's disease, Hodgkin's disease, multiple sclerosis, lupus, and ALS. The doctor said, "Your arm is not presenting the way I want, but I can't find anything specific." Funny thing is that I remember glancing through a pamphlet for ALS that day in the waiting room. I thought it was the most depressing thing I'd ever read. Nothing clicked about the symptoms it described.

On March 25, two months later, the specialist called us back in. He said, "I know I told you back in January that I couldn't find anything. Well, I was wrong." He went on to say: "You should quit your job; you need to convert your house or move; you have less than two years; there's not really a regime of drugs that will help because this is terminal." All the while he was talking, he never looked at me. Who did he think was going to look after this man?

His parting words were, "I can see this is a lot to take in. I'll call you in a couple of days." He never called. From that point on, we were flying blind in a frightening world. The doctor didn't even give us that horrible pamphlet.

We would see this doctor twice a year. My husband, fighting so hard to continue to work, to be useful, to participate in activities with family and friends, would look forward to these visits. He wanted his efforts to be recognized. All the doctor needed to say was something like, "Gosh, you're hanging in there so well—good for you." Instead, all he said was, "You're about where I expected you to be." And, as always, he never talked to me.

How could he say, "You're about where I expected you to be?" He had told us my husband would be dead in two years. In fact, he lived for almost six years, was sick only twice, and missed only one week of work in all that time. He worked until a Monday and died on a Wednesday. Imagine, "You're about where I expected you to be!" He had no idea what we were going through.

The only time this specialist ever acknowledged me on our twice yearly visits was when he could no longer understand what my husband was saying. He turned to me to ask me to interpret.

I couldn't resist what I did. I'd been leafing through a magazine, listening carefully to everything that was being said but in the posture of one who is being ignored. When the doctor spoke to me, I looked up with the look of someone who has been disturbed from a good read and said, "Oh, sorry, were you speaking to me?"

As we scanned our universe for anything that could help us, we found a group at the local rehab hospital. This was great for a while because they had a program in the pool to help reduce the stiffness in my husband's joints. Unfortunately, everyone else in the group died, and so the program was discontinued. I guess the fact that my husband was still alive didn't constitute a group!

We found the most useful information through the Internet, where we found an ALS group and could talk to both caregivers and patients from around the world. For example, when my husband started to choke, people online told us he needed a feeding tube. No one had suggested that we could be proactive. I still recall the day my husband sent me an email saying he was losing sensation in his tongue. This was a man who loved food. The move to the feeding tube was huge.

One of the best tips I got from this group was to use a condom as a urinary leg bag. As my husband became incontinent, he was involuntarily wetting his pants. Without the tip about the condom, we would have had to use diapers right away.

I also learned some tricks for moving my husband. No one had told me how to lift him into his wheelchair or onto the toilet or a shower bench. I used to joke that I was training for the Olympics in the clean, snatch, and jerk events.

This group was not only informative but also very supportive. I found out I wasn't the only person who dropped her husband on the floor. In fact, I could even share some tips from my own experience. For example, one night, when I tried to get my husband out of his chair without taking his socks off first, his feet just slid across the floor, and we both slowly went down. Everyone heard that one and the significance of socks!

The other great tip I got was that antidepressants help dry up saliva. My family doctor got a prescription for us that was such a help. Because my husband's tongue and throat muscles weren't working any longer to swallow saliva, he had been drooling constantly.

We had to go to the emergency room a couple of times. I've never seen such an overworked and compassionate group in my life as the staff in emergency! They always asked how I was doing, which was more than the specialist did!

The only other person who asked about me was my family doctor. She was fabulous, not just because she showed concern for me but because she'd get things for us and would follow up on things that had fallen through the cracks. She would also sometimes call us at home to see how we were doing.

By comparison, our regular appointments with the specialist were useless. We would ask questions about new drugs or treatments we had heard about, but all the doctor would say was, "You seem more versed than me on this one." We were always ahead of anything the formal system offered us. He never visited us and didn't even come to see my husband when he had to go to the hospital.

Do I sound like I was an angry caregiver? Well, I was. My husband knew this and didn't mind. He called me the "family ventilation system." I guess I would blow off steam for everyone.

For the most part, I felt I was on my own. We had great friends, some of whom cooked for us and made the kids' Christmas cookies so that they'd feel just like other kids when they took their lunches to school, and many of whom would come and sit with my husband and watch TV with him. But that just meant I could drive the kids to hockey games or music lessons or cook dinner. I needed a break, too. I was trying to be the family glue, maintain the semblance of ordinary life for everyone, and still go to work myself.

A regular day for me would involve getting up early to get my husband ready for work and the kids ready for school. Then I'd take my husband to work, go to work myself, pick up my husband for lunch and get him back to work again, go back to work myself, go back to get my husband, and be home for the kids after school. Then there were all the things that normally happen in a home with young children—homework, activities, a meal, bedtime—and then getting my husband ready for bed.

And nighttime was no picnic. I would have given almost anything for a full night's sleep. My husband described it best when he said, "On a good night, I only wake my wife up eight to ten times. On a bad night, it's every five minutes!"

I often wondered, "How long can I do this?" I felt so alone at night. When I was in the thick of things, I didn't have time to think. The feelings of isolation and exhaustion would come in the middle of the night.

Sometimes I'd just go into the bathroom and sit on the floor and have a good cry. I could only take a couple of minutes, though, and then I was back in action.

How did I look after myself? I didn't! I existed on pure adrenalin. I put on thirty-five pounds and remember thinking, *How did that happen? I didn't even have time to eat!*

Did I have any heroes? Friends, my family doctor, the staff in emergency, and two nurses stand out. The encounters were brief but brilliant!

In the first instance, in the fall of 2001, we made a heroic effort to travel up to Toronto for the Vanier Cup, which is the biggest football game of the year in the world of university football. When we got there, my husband's feeding tube was clogged. We mobilized, making a call to the city's special taxi service and heading to a downtown hospital. Once there, we heard, "Oh, we can't get to that until tomorrow—he'll have to stay overnight." I couldn't believe my ears . . . all this way to sit in a hospital? An older nurse overheard what was going on and said, "Does anyone have fifty cents? Go buy a can of Coke!" Ten minutes later, the Coke had cleared the feeding tube and we were on our way. My husband's team won and the players presented him with the trophy.

The second nurse worked on an inpatient unit. It was one of the two times my husband actually had to be in the hospital during the five and a half years of treatment. He was in a four-bed room. The patient who had been in bed three died, and the resident doctor wanted my husband moved to bed three, maybe because it was a bit nearer the door. I overheard this nurse, outside the door to our room, take on the doctor and say, "No he's not going to bed three. He knows someone just died in that bed, and he might think that's the 'dying bed.' He's going to stay where he is. A new patient can go to bed three." The doctor started to challenge her, but she just cut him off, saying, "Listen, you young pup. You can write me up if you like, but he is not going to bed three." Bravo! She deserved an Academy Award for best performance in a supporting role!

My kids? They were four and six when my husband got sick. They missed out on a lot—not only their dad, but time I couldn't spend with them. In a way, my kids are only now meeting the real me. My son, now fourteen, jokes with his friends, saying, "Great! I hit my teenage years, and my mom has time for me!"

My son and I have been in therapy for the last year. He had a lot of anger that I didn't tell him his father was sick and was going to die. We got his diagnosis in March and just wanted a couple of months to digest the information and figure out how we were going to go forward with all this, but the press got hold of the story. Because my husband had a high profile in the community, it became headline news without our knowing. Some kid came up to my son at school and said, "I'm sorry your dad is going to die." My husband's father found out on a bus when he saw it in the newspaper. What was news for the media turned out to be agony for us.

My daughter seems to be okay. She doesn't really remember a time when her dad wasn't sick. His changes over the five and a half years of treatment were gradual, and she seemed to adjust on a day-by-day basis.

What would I like to tell doctors? I want them to know that a terminal illness affects the entire family and that the entire family needs support.

Two years after my husband's death, I made an appointment to see the specialist who followed his case. I was in his office for an hour and just unloaded. I wanted him to know that he had ignored me and what that had felt like; that he had offered us virtually nothing at a time when we needed some sort of support and survival guide along with referrals to relevant resources; that he had no idea what we had to deal with on a day-to-day level; that the system had left us to fly blind; that it wasn't enough for a doctor to be smart—that social skills matter too. I wanted him to know that seeing a doctor every six months wasn't often enough—the changes with ALS are too dramatic and too fast for that. We needed to know that someone was on our team figuring out the plays before we got tackled. I told him that we had discovered the online group on our own—couldn't he have told us about that?

I described our experience of being seen in a clinic in another city in which all the relevant specialists saw the patients with ALS and came up with coordinated suggestions from various care specialties. I explained that while the patients were being seen, the family members got to meet together and find out what others were doing to manage, to cope. I added that, while at this clinic, we were given a book called the *ABCs of ALS*. I asked him why there couldn't be something like that here, especially given that we had the highest per-capita incidence of ALS and multiple sclerosis in the whole country.

Did this meeting make me feel better? Yes, especially when I started to hear from others in our community who had ALS and were served by the same specialist. Apparently, this doctor has changed and is now paying attention and relating to people in ways that feel very human. This is a good beginning.

Living the Opposites

Jane is bright, articulate, funny, active, and strong. At age fifty-five, she swims fifty laps every weekday, walks ten kilometers every weekend, and runs a large arts organization with an infectious passion. Jane's strength is not only physical (she has been known to crack ribs with her enthusiastic hugs) but also psychological (she can handle a lot of tough stuff). Jane was diagnosed with multiple sclerosis twenty-four years ago, breast cancer five years ago, and a troubling heart condition two years ago.

Jane points to a sign over her desk. It says "No Sniveling." "That's my approach to most things," she says. "I don't feel sick and I'm not into being sick. It's tedious, boring, and slows you down. I have no pain, no shortness of breath, no fatigue. I do have hot flashes from tamoxifen, but so what? That's no big deal."

Five years ago, Jane had not been feeling well, had found a lump in her breast, and had gone through a series of tests. At 4 p.m. on Christmas Eve, she received the news that she had breast cancer. A mastectomy revealed that twenty of twenty-four lymph nodes examined also were affected. She was referred to the Cancer Care Clinic to learn about her treatment options and was encouraged to bring someone with her to the consultation. Jane took a friend. She tells her story this way:

> Every step along the way, people were kindness person-
> ified. At that first consultation, I was scheduled for half
> an hour, but the doctor spent two and a half hours with
> us. He outlined a number of options, drew pictures,
> showed us graphs, explained procedures, and then said,
> "Now I'm going to leave you for half an hour so the two
> of you can talk without me here. When I come back, I'd

like you to tell me what your preliminary decision is for which option you want to follow. It's only preliminary because you can change your mind during the coming week, but it will help us all start to focus on what's best for you." Brilliant! He gave us clear information, then space and time alone, all with no pressure.

I have nothing but praise for the Cancer Care Clinic. I could call night or day. The nurses were angels. I went through radiation and chemotherapy. It was positive, positive, positive. I felt blessed, but then I entered an entirely different world.

Because I am taking tamoxifen and a possible side effect can be cancer of the cervix, I promised to have regular Pap smears. But you know how life is—you get busy, you feel healthy, you forget. Three years into taking tamoxifen, I finally booked an appointment through my family doctor. I was a bit surprised that even though I called for an appointment in November, I couldn't get an appointment until January. Surprise turned to concern when the appointment was rebooked three times. But concern turned to irritation when I showed up for my appointment at 7 a.m. and waited until 8:30, and still my doctor had not arrived. That's when I left and turned my irritation into action into getting a new family doctor.

My new doctor, a tiny, wee woman who looked like a kid, was fabulous. I had my first full visit with her in early March 2004. In addition to doing the Pap test, she listened to my heart and lungs and took my blood pressure. "How long have you had a heart murmur?" she asked. "And how long have you had high blood pressure?"

My blood pressure was 170/128. This was news to me because my previous doctor had never taken it. She never told me about any heart murmur either. It was Friday.

This new doctor scheduled me for an electrocardiogram (ECG) on Monday. The technicians repeated the ECG three times, telling me that they thought their machines were broken. Then they asked me to wait while they faxed the results to my doctor. She called me while I was still in the ECG room and said, "The ECG says you're having a heart attack, and I want you to go to the emergency room right away."

When I arrived in emergency, I discovered that if you have my kind of ECG slip, you get seen right away and get hooked up to lots of machines. The doctors and nurses were all shaking their heads as they looked at the jagged lines on the machines and asked, sounding skeptical, "You really swim fifty laps every day?"

The emergency doctors said I should get more tests, but four months passed and I heard nothing. Didn't bother me, really, because I had no symptoms, but I called my new family doctor to tell her that nothing had been scheduled. She made a couple of calls. Tests were scheduled.

What I remember most about that series of tests is that when I was on the treadmill, I never got tired. And yet, the technicians said things like, "Oh my god, can you feel that? Your heart is doing funny things." I found their comments somewhat alarming, but I didn't feel anything.

Next, I had a twenty-four-hour heart-monitor test. I was told it would take three weeks to get the results. After four weeks, I called. A receptionist told me I wouldn't hear for another two months. And that's when I started to make calls, leaving messages for the cardiologist, trying to sound like a squeaky wheel or a dying duck or a pathetic version of *Swan Lake*. Turns out, the results of the twenty-four-hour trace had been lost and I would have to repeat the test.

I got a message on Friday to show up for the test on Monday at 9 a.m. On Monday, I sat there until noon. I asked the nurse, "Is the doctor here, ill, or somewhere else?" She said, "I'll page him," and then left for lunch.

The doctor showed up at 1:15 p.m. I'd never met him before, but his first words were, "How are you, dear?" I started to get mad, but then I laughed. It was all so ridiculous! I explained that I'd had all sorts of tests because there was something about my heart that seemed to be alarming to doctors. This all had started in March, it was now September, and I really had no idea what was going on.

This doctor was ultimately able to tell me what was wrong structurally with my heart (ventricular tachycardia) and suggested that I have a catheterization to find the specific locus of the problem. Seemed like a plan.

In mid-October, I went into the hospital on a Wednesday night to be monitored for thirty-six hours. The procedure was going to be on Friday morning. I was sharing the room with a woman who was very sick and in a lot of pain. It can't have been any fun for her because I kept setting the monitors off at the nursing station and the nurses would run in every twenty minutes to see if I was okay.

My cardiologist had said he'd be in on Friday morning at 7 a.m. to go over everything with me. By 8:30, a group of doctors (without mine, though) came in on rounds. My case was clearly interesting to them because it was so bizarre, but they talked among themselves as though I wasn't there. One doctor in the group was very opposed to the procedure I was about to have, believing it to be dangerous and clinically inappropriate.

Although I appreciate that it's important for doctors to give patients a full spectrum of information about treatment options, having a disagreement in front of me, without involving me, is just not acceptable. You already feel very vulnerable when you're ill. The doctors' argument was extremely frightening and I just lost it. I started shouting at them, screaming, and then I burst into tears. My roommate applauded as the doctors scurried out of my room.

My doctor finally showed up and calmed me down. By then, however, it was too late to do the procedure and it had to be rebooked for two weeks later. And I'm supposed to be avoiding stress!

Then it was early November, and I was actually in the operating room, prepped and waiting for surgery. It was determined that there was still one more consent form I had to sign. And, believe it or not, the same guy who had been so opposed to the procedure two weeks before was the one who brought me the papers, and he was still trying to persuade me not to go ahead! I told him to "just scram and stop messing with my head." I had more important things to focus my energy on at the moment.

I was awake for the whole procedure. It normally takes two to three hours; mine lasted for more than eight hours. But it seemed to work, and the pictures they took the next morning looked like a normal heart. The doctors said they'd follow up with me in January. In April, I called them.

Two weeks later, I did the halter monitor thing, and ten days after that, on a Friday afternoon, I reported in to get the results. Another hour and a half wait and a new doctor came in saying, "What are you here for?" I told him I was tired of people not knowing who I was or what was going on. We ended up looking through the file together and found the test results. My heart was again behaving as it had before the surgery. I had to have another stress test.

I've now had that test, and, once again, I haven't heard the results. I'm still hanging and I don't like hanging. I'm not easily frightened and I'm not afraid to die, but this current situation—the not knowing—is stressful and I don't need it! I have a life to live.

I know doctors are busy and I try to cut them some slack, but I have a life, too. The doctors may not think I am as important as they are, but my view is that everyone is equally important. And I'm especially important to me. I just want to be treated as a thinking human being who has a full and complex life.

As a cancer patient and as a cardiology patient, I feel I've been on different planets. But this means I know what's possible. I've experienced how it can be. I've lived the opposites.

The Journey of the Green Elephant

The coffee cup rests on a side table. On closer examination, the table is, in fact, an elegant green porcelain elephant. The woman opposite notices my gaze, sinks back into a comfortable, stuffed armchair, and travels back in time. She begins speaking.

Great Care and Great Love

It took me a year to pick up that elephant and bring him home. It's a long story.

I was twenty-eight, in New York on a business trip, and had bought a beautiful, thigh-high, green ceramic elephant at an art gallery the day before. I remember calling my mother and saying, "I feel like I'm on top of the world. I have just picked out a wonderful new piece of art, and I love my job and I feel great!" At the time, I was unmarried and working in Toronto as a lawyer.

The next day I had a terrible attack of pain while walking down Madison Avenue. I staggered into some little restaurant, draped myself over a table, and waited for the pain to subside. When I got home, I experienced a similar attack but this time had to go to the bathroom. When I looked in the toilet bowl, I gasped because my stools were bright, emerald green. I went to my doctor right away. She gave me a stool test kit and said to return with the testing complete. I never made it back.

By early the next morning, pain was gripping my neck, chest, and side. I also felt like I was choking. A friend drove me to the hospital, and I remember urging him to go through the red lights. I knew I had to get help right away. I collapsed in the entrance to emergency. I heard someone yelling, "No BP. No pulse."

The next thing I remember is being on a stretcher that was being pushed very quickly down a hallway. A doctor, running alongside of me, said, "We're taking you into surgery. You're bleeding inside." I could see bags and bags of blood on some kind of dress rack near me. It was the beginning of the AIDS scare. I looked hazily at him and said, "I'm going to get AIDS!" He replied, "Lady, that's the least of your concerns."

I heard that the doctor got into trouble for what he said, but I think he saved my life. There was something about his intensity and seriousness that made me click into survival mode. My mind whispered, "Pamela—participate!" This I did as much as I could from then on. I knew I had to participate to live, to keep my soul in my body.

I was on the operating table for more than fifteen hours. It turned out I had a hepatic adenoma, which is a single-cell, benign tumor. It had exploded and blown my liver and gall bladder into pieces. Following the resection of my liver, apparently I kept bleeding out. While the team of surgeons tried to stabilize me, a determined hematologist kept trying to mix potions for me in his lab. He wouldn't quit. Thank heaven!

Of course, I was told about the medical facts of this very long day only much later. Some of the details I heard paralleled what I had experienced in another dimension. I recall two images of my dying.

During the first, I was in a stream of warm air and floating away from my body. I saw my dead grandmother and told her, "I'm not ready yet." I turned my back against the flow of the warm air, but I still wanted to talk to her. Over my shoulder, I said, "I'm sorry they didn't let me go to your funeral." She replied, "Darling, I've always known. Now go." And then I literally dove back into my body, comforted by an image of friends and family waiting for me.

Some time passed, and I sensed I couldn't hold on any longer. I felt like horses were pounding me and I had to let go. At the last minute, I had the sensation of someone pinning me in my body and I thought, *He's holding me. I have to stay.*

When I came to, I saw my parents. They'd flown halfway across the country when they heard I'd been taken into emergency and had collapsed. I moved my left hand in circles and my father took that to mean that I wanted a pen. I wrote, "Thanks for coming." As soon as he saw me include the period, my dad said he knew I'd be okay. I never saw his optimism crack.

A week and half later, there was a new emergency. My bile duct was leaking. I had to go back to surgery and be opened up again. A few weeks later, I needed a third surgery because necrotic liver tissue was festering inside me. This time, they went in through the back, and my doctor had to remove a rib to be able to properly clean out my thoracic cavity. The space where my rib had been was packed and bandaged.

My doctor was going away for a couple of days, which made me nervous. He assured me I'd be okay and that he'd remove the packing when he came back. He specifically told me not to let anyone take it out until he got back.

Two days later, Halloween to be exact, when my father was downstairs getting a cup of coffee and I was alone in my room, the senior surgical resident came in. He told me he was going to remove the packing from my wound. I remembered my doctor's admonition to keep the packing in and my internal voice that had said "participate"! I explained that Doctor T. had said he didn't want the packing removed and that he'd do it when he returned. The resident's response was, "Well, he's away and I'm in charge." He turned me over, removed the packing, then left my room.

I drifted off. Then I opened my eyes and saw that my entire bed was covered in blood. I was so weak I couldn't reach the call button. When my father came back to my room, he dropped his coffee and ran for the nurses. In the chaos that followed, my feeding tube also got dislodged. I remember general pandemonium . . . people running and others appearing out of nowhere . . . people calling things out to me, to someone. The chaos made me panic. I started to hyperventilate.

The senior surgical resident came back in and was yelling his name at me and telling me to calm down. Seeing him made me panic more. Another resident, Jacques-who-I'll-never-forget, told me to look into his eyes and breathe into a paper bag. He was my friend. He used to come and tell me about his life. I knew him enough to trust him and calm down. The bleeding was staunched, but I had to have several transfusions.

When my doctor returned, he was furious. It turned out he hadn't wanted the packing removed because I was on a blood thinner and he knew that would have to be stopped first. The senior resident came in to apologize, but I couldn't look at him. I was afraid of him from then on.

My father held me together that day. The only thing I had from home was a beautiful blue bathrobe. When I saw that it was also soaked in blood, I felt something inside me dissolve. I said to my father, "Daddy, I don't think I can master this. This is too much for us to handle." His response: "We can handle anything. Don't worry. I guarantee you'll feel better after a couple of hours of sleep." Comforted by his reassurance, I succumbed to my exhaustion. It had been a messy Halloween.

When I woke up, it was barely dawn. I saw my father in the armchair beside my bed and asked him if he'd been there all night. "No," he said, "I went home for a bit." He paused and then said, "I have something for you." And he handed me my bathrobe . . . as clean, clear, and blue as a summer sky, fresh and perfectly ironed. He'd gone home to wash it and was seen ironing it at 5 a.m. There was no residue of any mayhem anywhere I looked. He was drinking his morning coffee. The sun was up. We were fine.

Both of my parents took exquisite, intuitive care of my sense of self, how I viewed my situation, how it all looked from the inside out. My frame of mind was one thing they could actively manage. The bathrobe was important and symbolic to me and so it was to my dad. My physical sense of self was shocked and fragile, and my mother tended to it as she would a newborn.

After the second surgery, two nurses came in to change my dressings and one said to my mother, "It's pretty gruesome. You may want to step outside." I said, "It's okay, Mom. You can come right back after. You don't have to watch." But my mother just looked at me and said, "If you're staying, I'm staying. If I love you, I love your wounds." My long, deep, open wounds never seemed worrisome again, at least not to me.

My parents were a seamless blend of strength and optimism. Their love for me kept me alive as I faced a long tunnel of darkness. Their devotion held me as if transfixed on the path home.

Over ten or twelve weeks, nurses came and went, but there seemed to be too many other lives and deaths around our floor for them to connect to anyone. They told me stories about the guy next door, and then he died. And then more stories about another guy, and then he died. I'm not sure who needed the distance between us more, the nurses or me.

One thing that was memorable was a pending nurses' strike,

which made matters worse. One nurse said, "You're a lawyer. I'm sure you understand our concerns. We just have to strike." But her words struck cold fear into me. All I could understand, lawyer or not, was that her serious and dire concerns did not include my welfare in any way. I was hooked up to machines and completely dependent on the hospital staff to live, but I was not on her mind at all. I was petrified. All I could think of was, *If there's a strike, what's going to happen to me?*

I have fond memories of two residents who connected with me as a real person. They'd drop in, ask me how I was doing, and just chat. For example, one of them described his daughter's bumblebee costume that she'd be wearing for Halloween. The other one, Jacques-who-I'll-never-forget, told me about taking someone on a date to see a movie and what the movie had been like. These conversations helped me remember there was a real world out there where people did normal things. These chats linked me to a life I could have beyond the hospital.

Several months after collapsing in emergency, and three operations later, I was scarred, covered in bandages, and incredibly weak, but well enough to go home to recuperate.

My surgeon said, "I want to ask you something unorthodox. There's a whole team of people who have been quietly cheering for you since the first dark days. They want to see you going home, and I want you to meet them." I was dressed to leave the hospital, and so he wheeled me down to the surgical staff lounge. There were about thirty-five people there, waiting for me. They began clapping and cheering for me. I was dumbfounded. I clapped back to them. I started to cry. Some of them also cried.

My surgeon had been fantastic. He had showed tremendous respect for me as a person. He always made me feel like he spent his whole morning getting ready to see me. Every time I saw him, he'd say, "How's my fighter?" I felt we were partners together in a project and neither of us would let the other down. I certainly would not be letting him down.

I am sure I survived only because of my doctor's great care and my parents' great love. None of them ever let me believe that something couldn't be handled. All three of them were my partners. My parents were also my guardians and my advocates. My doctor was my champion.

"Creepy"

After a month at home, it was time to start rehab. Everyone called me "Creepy" because of how I walked. I couldn't stand up straight and could only shuffle my feet. All the bed rest in the hospital had created a scoliosis in my spine.

I went to rehab every day for five hours, for six months. There were times they would have me do something, such as climb up a couple of steps and down again, and I'd have to have a nap. Everything was so tough. Small bags of peanuts were the first weights I lifted.

My mother drove me to rehab every morning at 9:30 and picked me up every afternoon. In the car one day, I remember saying, "I can't go there again. I can't do this again. How am I going to get through this? What am I going to do?" And she said, "You just open the door. You just go in. I love you. I have nothing else to say." It must have been so difficult for her to see me working so hard and still struggling so much. She was my rock, and she was steadfast with her love, her support, and her focus. And, of course, I knew what I had to do: "Pamela—participate."

After the six months of rehab, I had regained some strength and some flexibility, but I was not finished. I still had more hurdles to clear.

Maimonides' Prayer

Ten months after my initial emergency collapse, it was determined that I was ready to talk about future reconstructive surgery on my abdomen. It felt really important to me to check out the prospect of minimizing the disfigurement I had suffered. I knew I would need to have some muscles and ribs rearranged, and I also needed some plastic surgery to diminish the magnitude and lumpiness of some very long, very deep, puffy scars, almost like trenches, running at angles deep into my trunk.

I was referred to someone described as the "most famous and very best" plastic surgeon in the country. I can't even begin to describe how excited I was to be traveling fifteen hundred miles to see this doctor. The fact that I was now well enough to take this trip by myself was huge. And this artist genius was going to put me back into a young woman's body.

At the time, I was thin and pale, and my hair was short. Much of my hair had fallen out in the hospital and was just growing back. Because of my extensive scarring, I couldn't tuck any clothes into my waist, but I dressed up as much as I could. I can still see myself. I wore a big white shirt of my father's and flowery pants with a loose waist.

The plastic surgeon's office was unlike any I'd ever seen. Tastefully decorated, it had sophisticated furniture, soft classical music, and a wall fountain. I'd never seen one before. I was in a complete state of awe and excited anticipation.

A nurse took me into an interior office. She told me to get undressed, wrap a sheet around myself, and stand up on the footstool in the middle of the room. When the doctor came in, he told me to drop the sheet. He circled around me, asking questions and nodding. Then he stopped, looked at me (the sheet was still on the floor), and said, "I could make you look once again like a beautiful, young woman; I could fix you, but I won't. Your case is covered by medical insurance and the insurance doesn't pay me enough to keep my children in private schools."

A chasm opened up inside of me. I felt I was falling into it. My eyes brimmed with tears. I had to get away from there. As I stood there, completely naked, he said I was not worth his effort.

Subdued and shaken, I got dressed and began to leave his office. As I reached the door, the doctor looked up from his desk, where two ivory tusks on the wall behind him framed him. He asked how I had heard of him. I replied that he had been recommended by my cousin, Dr. X, a physician in the same city. He suddenly became interested and said, "Oh, your cousin is Dr. X? Well, perhaps we should talk." I was incredulous. I knew that I wanted nothing to do with this man.

Many years after this event, my father-in-law quoted a man named Maimonides, who lived in the twelfth century. He was a scholar, philosopher, codifier of laws, and a very thoughtful and famous physician. Maimonides' "Prayer of the Physician" says:

"O Lord . . . Preserve me from the temptation of allowing myself to be influenced in the exercise of my profession by the thirst for gain or the pursuit of glory. Strengthen my heart so that it may be ever ready to serve both poor and rich, both friend and foe, both just and unjust."

My guess is that Maimonides would have been very disappointed by the famous plastic surgeon and my encounter with him.

I Think of That Nurse Every Day

Months later, I was referred to another plastic surgeon. He was extremely competent and very kind. Based on my previous experience, I'd say I actually ended up with the best after all. He even gave me a belly button again.

After the corrective surgery, my doctor left detailed instructions for the nursing staff. He also told me how the bandages that encased my entire torso should be wrapped when the dressings were changed. He was very specific and insistent about the importance of the bandage not only covering my scars, but also that they come down a few inches below the scar line.

My first nurse followed the doctor's instructions and did it perfectly. Hours passed and there was a shift change.

Eventually, I realized my dressings were overdue to be changed. I buzzed for the nurse and asked if they could be done. The new nurse had a chip on her shoulder. Assuming I was in the hospital for a tummy tuck, she said, "I know you're a cosmetic patient—I'll get to you when I get to you."

When this nurse finally did come in, she was cold and nasty and she bound me incorrectly, not taking the bandage down far enough. I asked her if she could please fully cover the scar. I explained that my doctor had been very explicit about how it should be done. She challenged me, saying, "Are you telling me how to do my job? I don't have time to do this again. There are people here with real injuries. My priority is not your tummy tuck."

I was shocked! I was rendered mute by both her callousness and by the worrisome realization that she had worked on me without really reading the chart.

Because of that nurse, I have an ugly bump on my belly, beneath the scars crisscrossing my body. The scars remind me of excellent care and a life saved. The red bump reminds me of someone's bad mood and disdain. I think of that nurse every day. I wish I'd been more forceful with her.

I believe that when you are dealing with an unpleasant sales-clerk at a department store, you're actually in training for the occasional health care professional who seems to be missing the empathy gene. Fortunately, they are in the minority, and I do have faith in the system as a whole.

From Being Healed to Being Saved

While recuperating at home, I saw my family doctor regularly. He would check my progress and sometimes we'd just talk. On one visit, I told him, "I think there's something wrong with my face. It feels a bit paralyzed." He replied that it could be some residual nerve damage, given everything I'd been through, but asked me to tell him again how it felt. I said, "It feels like I have a mask on my face."

He said, "I think you're in a depression. And if anyone has reason for a depression, it would be you. I recommend that you see Dr. Y, a psychiatrist. I think the two of you will have a lot to talk about."

My sessions with Dr. Y were completely liberating. I went through every step of my ordeal with him. I came to under-stand that I was suffering from post-traumatic stress, something unheard of twenty years ago. I had badly needed to talk about what had happened to me but hadn't wanted to share the details of the awfulness with the people I loved. I had created a protective mask.

This skillful psychiatrist guided me through the last steps of my journey, past being physically healed to being psychologically saved.

·····

After five hours, our conversation comes to a natural close. The green elephant sits there, quietly, as though watching her, bearing witness, having taken everything in.

This woman fully recovered and returned to work. She is now married, has four children and a warm and nourishing home, and has started a school based on "awe and wonder." She is also a talented artist, and the images in her paintings are bold and strong. Her memories of her previous health care experiences, albeit still vivid, are just memories, not daily challenges. Daily challenges now include helping with homework, renovating a house, and finding time as a hospital board member to read a report on "enhancing the quality of patient care."

I Needed a Guide

It was a warm August night. It should have been perfect for the fireworks display scheduled to celebrate the city's birthday, but heavy fog had moved in from the harbor, settling in, obscuring the view. The crowds of people began to disperse.

Beth, a single mother, began to walk to the car with her two sons and a couple of children from her neighborhood. Beth's husband, the boys' father, was not there. Richard, an emergency room physician and orthopedic surgeon, had died a year earlier as a result of liver cancer.

There were hundreds of people about, all moving toward cars and home. Several were crossing a wide boulevard using the pedestrian crosswalk. Then there was a terrible sound—a thud— the sound of a car connecting with a human body. Beth's younger son, Adam, had been hit by a car traveling too fast. The driver was oblivious to the crowds of people and to the crosswalk sign. The driver was oblivious because the driver was drunk.

The ambulance arrived before Beth knew it, and her son was sped off to the hospital, with Beth following behind in a police car. Paul, Adam's brother and Beth's older son, was to go to a friend's house and wait for her there.

At the hospital, a social worker greeted Beth as she walked through the door. In Beth's words, "This was the most important element of the care I received at the hospital." She continues:

> Hospitals are very strange places under the best of cir-
> cumstances. In a serious emergency situation, you need
> a guide. You're in shock and need handholding, some-
> one to help your mind work, to see what you can do
> and then help you do it. You basically need to borrow

a working mind. You have to make decisions. Someone has to help you see what decisions are to be made. This social worker filled this need for me. She had lost family, too, and she understood. Not only was she a godsend that night, but she also stayed in touch with me for several weeks, which was a comfort.

The second most important need Beth had was for information. She desperately wanted to know what was going on. She did know that Adam had been taken immediately to the operating room, but that was all she knew. As it turned out, a friend, an orthopedic surgeon who just happened to be in the hospital that night, facilitated communication between the operating room and the small private room where Beth was waiting.

This friend was able to give Beth an indication that things were not going well. It helped, she said, to have some warning of the cruel reality that was to follow. "My mind had been fighting against the worst possibilities. I'd been thinking we could go home soon. I realized I needed to shift my thinking and to get ready for the truth—that we wouldn't be going home, that Adam would never be coming home."

Beth had a very strong network of family and friends. Because there was a phone in the room where she was waiting, she was able to call people, to put them on alert, to ask them for help, to find out where her other son was, and to begin to make arrangements when the final, tragic truth of Adam's death was finally relayed to her.

The physician who had been in the operating room desperately trying to save Adam's life offered to speak to Beth's son Paul at any time. He knew that Paul might want or need to try to piece together what happened after his brother had been rushed away in the ambulance.

The guidance of the social worker and her follow-up calls, the communication flow to ease the burden of waiting in ignorance or in fantasy, the support of friends, and the offers for follow-up conversations kept Beth going. She says, "I do not know how awful this horrific situation would be for someone who is not in her hometown or for someone who speaks another language or for someone who is socially isolated."

· · · · ·

Beth had to endure reliving this trauma through the court case that ensued. The driver of the car that hit and killed Adam was found to be guilty of driving under the influence of alcohol. Beth and Paul have both spoken publicly about the powerful effects of combining alcohol and driving.

Rise & Shine

In early April, my wife, Bertha, had a biopsy of a breast lump that had come and gone for several months. Its erratic nature, combined with delays in the medical system, meant that Bertha kept missing the window for testing. After the biopsy was done, we were told that if there was a problem, we'd hear in two or three days. It was really hard to focus. We were both like robots at work, there in body but not in mind. At home, we'd often just wander around the house. We tried to distract ourselves with novels but couldn't concentrate.

We were on pins and needles for the first seventy-two hours, but, as the days passed without a phone call, we both began to relax. We presumed everything was okay. We noticed that the sun was shining again.

On April 20, Bertha went to our regular family doctor for a routine appointment. Because there was no reason to do otherwise, I didn't go with her. She went alone.

When Bertha walked into the doctor's office, at the beginning of the appointment, her doctor handed her a brochure titled, "How to Deal with Breast Cancer." Bertha read between the lines immediately. Obviously, a phone call that should have been made in the initial seventy-two hours after the biopsy had somehow been overlooked. Our family doctor, thinking he was being helpful, with a simple gesture, had pulled the ground out from under our feet.

The implied news that the lump had been malignant was completely unanticipated. Of course, Bertha was devastated. And when I finally found out what had happened, I was overcome not just with fear, but also with an enormous sense of guilt that Bertha had had to hear this news alone. I should have been with her!

As Bertha tried to absorb the fact that she had breast cancer and had to have surgery, I felt completely helpless. I felt the very center of our lives being threatened. There was only the tiniest sense of comfort that Bertha was going to get the medical help she needed. Quite legitimately, Bertha was being treated as the patient, but I felt I was also caught in the whirlwind of this terrifying illness. I needed to know what I could do. I needed a meaningful role to play. None was suggested by any doctor.

After Bertha's surgery, while waiting for her chemotherapy to begin, an idea began to form in my mind. I thought Bertha needed a smile, even if just for a second, and so I began to search through books for special sayings or quotations that might boost her spirits. It became a way for me to help her, to give her some encouragement, to say "you can do this!"

Bertha's chemotherapy started on June 10 and so did my found quotes—the first one was "Damn the torpedoes, full steam ahead!" (Admiral David Farragut). I always left the quotes on the kitchen table. I specifically left them there because it meant that Bertha had a reason to get out of bed each morning to see them. It gave her something to start her day.

I know they mattered to her. She said, in a recent speech she gave: "The quotes were a bright spot in my day. I'd stick them up all around the house—in the kitchen, in the bathroom, beside my pillow—wherever I might need some encouragement. I put some up beside my copy of *Warnings of Possible Reactions to Chemotherapy*. The quotes served as a countermeasure to the dreadful reality I was dealing with. Some of them are still up on my mirror even now. One can always use some motivation!"

These daily gifts to my beloved wife also helped me deal with my own private pain and agonizing sense of helplessness.

Through it all, I got the satisfaction that I was doing something. I was helping Bertha cope. It was no big deal, but it worked for both of us.

It doesn't make me any kind of hero. In fact, this whole cancer journey has changed my thoughts about heroes. I used to think that people like Winston Churchill were my heroes, but I've changed my view. It's the people on the cancer wards—the nurses, doctors, and pharmacists, and the women who are fighting breast cancer—they're my heroes now!

•••••

Bertha and her husband, Wayne, gave this collection of quotes to the Canadian Breast Cancer Foundation to use as a fundraiser and to boost the spirits of others who journey in crisis. The collection was published under the title of Rise & Shine. *A second volume of 180 quotes was released in2006. Bertha continues in remission, and Wayne hopes that a cure for breast cancer will be found.*

A Profoundly Isolating Experience

Maggie holds her coffee cup. She is simply and neatly dressed and she looks completely composed. She starts talking, in a calm, soft-spoken manner. It is clear she has given this interview a lot of thought. Her words come slowly, somewhat haltingly. And then she stops and apologizes for what she describes as "being so dumb." She adds, "I think I've processed all of this, but my hands are shaking."

She closes her eyes and rubs her temples and forehead, as if to carefully retrieve the ten-year journey of her husband's illness. It's been seven years since Richard died.

Before she goes any further, Maggie stresses that she does not want to name or blame. "I'm grateful to all the people who cared for Richard. They did the best they could. I know that all health care professionals mean well." She is so gracious and repeats this sentiment many times during the next two hours.

Richard's nosebleeds began in 1988, two and a half years after Maggie and Richard were married. At that time, they had a one-year-old, and Maggie was pregnant with their second child. They were living in a suburb of a large city, far away from both of their families.

Richard traveled a lot and thought that possibly his nosebleeds were being caused by the dry air of long airplane flights. One of his nosebleeds occurred while he was in Germany and was so bad he had to be hospitalized. The bleeding stopped and he was able to fly home, but he realized it was time to go see a doctor.

Richard ended up being referred to an ear, nose, and throat specialist. He didn't see any need for Maggie to come to his appointments with him. Initially, she didn't give this a second thought, in part because it would have been difficult with a one-year-old and no babysitter.

The specialist decided that Richard should have exploratory surgery to try to determine what was causing the nosebleeds. "Maybe Richard knew that the surgery was, in fact, a biopsy, but that word was never mentioned to me. Nonetheless, I wanted to be at the hospital when the doctor spoke to my husband about what he found during surgery. I couldn't contact the doctor at the hospital and so I kept calling his office to say—'I'm home with a young baby and can't wait at the hospital all day. Please just ask the doctor to let me know when he's going to talk to Richard and I can get there in thirty minutes.' "

Either the doctor never got the message or he didn't think it was important for Maggie to be there when he told Richard that surgery had revealed a cancerous mass that looked like adenoid cystic carcinoma.

Maggie did accompany Richard to a follow-up appointment with this doctor to learn about what was in store for her husband. The doctor walked into the office and said, "Hi Richard, would your wife mind leaving the room?"

Maggie recalls:

I can't believe it, but I did leave the room. I felt so angry and so vulnerable and so intimidated. I think the doctor just wanted a very clinical experience and was afraid I'd demonstrate some sort of emotion. But he didn't even know me. In fact, I hardly ever cry and never in public. He was shutting me out of my own life for reasons that weren't valid in my case.

Richard, too, kept a certain distance after the initial stage of treatment, saying he didn't need me to go to his appointments with him. I think he needed to feel some control when things were so out of control. Whenever I asked about the appointments, he didn't tell me very much. I was young, pregnant, and far away from family and friends. I couldn't get my questions answered directly by anyone.

Two weeks after the diagnosis, Richard was scheduled for surgery to remove the tumor. The operation was supposed to take place at 8 a.m., but the surgeon did not arrive until 2 p.m. By that time, Richard was not only hungry and impatient, but he'd also had a long time to think about his work and upcoming commitments. Apparently, he asked his surgeon if he would be able to attend a meeting in Toronto the following week.

Maggie learned about this because the same doctor who had asked her to leave his office ten days earlier now called her at home immediately after Richard's surgery. Maggie describes that he sounded furious as he said, "Your husband just asked me if he can travel next week. Clearly, you guys aren't taking this seriously. This isn't the flu. This will likely travel to his brain and kill him."

"That was all he said. I just looked at the phone after he hung up. There had been no kindness in his voice, only irritation. I had seen my grandfather die slowly, stroke after stroke, and I suddenly saw what was likely ahead of me. I kept this horrifying reality to myself. I never told anyone about the doctor's call."

For the next three years, Richard had lots of radiation and continued to work and go to his doctor's appointments alone. Any information Maggie had was through Richard, secondhand. Life just went on.

Then Maggie started to notice that one of Richard's eyes didn't look right. She'd tell Richard, "I think there's something different about your eye. Please tell your doctor that your wife is concerned and that she thinks you should have a CT scan. And Richard would come back from an appointment and say, 'The doctor thinks I only need one CT scan a year and I'm not scheduled for one for several months.' "

"No one was listening to my concerns, including Richard's ophthalmologist. Eventually, however, his eye looked so strange that anyone could tell from looking at him that something was terribly wrong." What happened next was a turning point for Maggie.

After nine months, Richard finally had his regularly scheduled CT scan. Maggie continues her story:

> The doctor called both of us in and told Richard, "You have a problem I can't deal with, and I'm going to refer you to a head and neck specialist." He gave us Richard's file to take to the new doctor. I read it from cover to cover, including the report from the radiologist that spelled out, in words even I could understand, that there was a huge and new tumor. Clearly, there'd been an unnecessary lag in diagnosis. You'd think an eye doctor would have been concerned that Richard's eye had been showing lots of vascular activity for months. And after three years of following Richard, this doctor didn't have the guts to tell us what had been found. He just passed us off.
>
> You want to believe that doctors will fix everything, but sometimes they're not paying attention or don't know or admit to the limitations of their own expertise.

I learned the hard way. It took this brutal experience to make me assert myself and get involved. I told Richard that I'd be coming to his appointments and that I'd be speaking up and that he needed to get ready.

We went to see the new head and neck doctor together. He was a kind, older man who told Richard, in complicated medical language, that the cancer had spread to his eye and would require surgery. Because I had lived with my sister, who is an orthoptist, I understood some "medicalese." I also knew from reading the file that Richard had had a recurrence and that when the doctors talked about "treatment," that meant that Richard would lose his eye. They were using such complex language, however, that Richard had to ask, "Will the surgery affect my eye?"

I concluded that it was this doctor's own humanity that kept him from spelling things out or preparing us for the tough realities we would be facing. It was as though he wanted to protect us and thought that if he just asked us how our Thanksgiving was and didn't tell us things, we wouldn't worry. I also think he was uncomfortable with the situation himself, but if you can't communicate bad news, then why go into medicine?

Richard's eye was removed. And over the following six years, he had nine more operations.

It was like my husband was chained to a radiator and couldn't escape the invisible monster living in the house who fed on Richard's flesh. The monster would come out now and then and take pieces of him, but the experts didn't want to talk to us about the situation. We wanted to know when the monster was likely to come out again, and how they would deal with it, but it was as though the doctors would merely say, "Don't worry! We're the monster tamers. We'll take care of everything."

Not having specific information did not keep me from worrying. If you don't know what to worry about specifically, then you worry about everything. My imagination worked overtime, especially at night. I conjured up horrible things and often felt like I was living out my nighttime fears during the day.

On top of everything else, our new baby had very bad asthma, the kind where they don't ask you for any information when you run into emergency room; they just grab your child and start treatment. At home, I had to give him medicine every four hours. I had to keep him alive. I didn't get enough sleep. I coped, but I was depressed. I shut down. In hindsight, I missed our baby's infancy.

Richard's surgeries left him horrifically disfigured. It was a profoundly isolating experience. I couldn't appreciate what it was like to be in Richard's shoes, he couldn't appreciate what it was like to be in my shoes, and no one could appreciate what it was like to be in our shoes.

Although Richard seemed to handle everything magnificently, we didn't really talk about things. It was only after he died, when I was going through all the papers in his desk, that I found something he'd written that conveyed how isolated he had felt.

Of course, the kids were affected by all this as well. Our baby, when he was two, drew pictures of eyes everywhere and would go around the house chanting, "First Daddy had two eyes, and then he had one." Our three-year-old understood that the doctors had used a knife to take his daddy's eye away and quietly concluded they could take everything away and that his dad could disappear completely.

I can't tell you how many times I felt like I was supposed to just sit in a corner like a golden retriever and smile. It was as though I was wallpaper. A group of physicians would come into a tiny examining room and introduce themselves to Richard and completely ignore me. I wanted to scream, "Didn't you have mothers? Weren't you taught manners?" I didn't scream, though, because I wanted the staff to like my husband. It was a difficult balancing act—"be nice, but make sure Richard gets what he needs."

There was a time when Richard was in a horrible state. By then I knew his situation so well I could tell he was facing a crisis and, if something wasn't done, he would die. His doctor had dismissed his problems as a cold. I took him to the emergency room and told the staff that he had to be seen and I wasn't going home. The doctors finally agreed that Richard's condition was not only serious, it was very grave. He needed major brain and facial reconstructive surgery. It took three days to put together a team of ten surgeons to perform the fourteen-hour operation.

I suppose this whole situation could have been intimidating, but I was beyond intimidation. I knew I had to do what I could to keep him alive. Richard wouldn't advocate for himself. I know that I saved his life that day by being so fierce.

When asked if there were any positive memories about Richard's care, Maggie immediately says:

Above all, I'm grateful for everything that everyone did. They gave us ten years, but there are three doctors who stand out, and two of them were part of the team who helped Richard through that particular crisis.

As each member of the team was found, the doctors, one by one, came in to meet Richard. One of them arrived a bit later than he'd said, and the first words out of his mouth were, "Sorry to keep you waiting." In ten years, he was the only one who ever said that! And when I asked him if he'd ever done this operation before, he didn't flinch from the question but spoke the truth. He said, "I've done a dozen other operations with this level of complexity, but I've never done exactly this. We'll be making this up as we go." I appreciated his honesty.

Another of the doctors came in and introduced himself to both of us (rare in itself). Then he asked Richard how old he was (thirty-seven), where he lived (a nearby suburb), and whether he had any children (two). Through these three simple questions, this doctor communicated that he understood there was a whole human being in the bed. I almost wept because this doctor was acknowledging his shared humanity with my husband. This was incredibly important to me at that time, and I'll never forget this man.

The third doctor who was special was the one Richard had during his last year. The doctor who had followed Richard for six years called us into his office and said, with tears in his eyes, "Go home and live your life." This was his way of saying, "There's nothing more to be done." We pressed for another answer, however, and ended up with a wonderful oncologist who bravely took on Richard's case. He always asked Richard, "What have you noticed?" Then he would ask me, too. He spoke clearly and honestly and with genuine kindness. He sought out treatment options and coordinated Richard's care. I no longer felt that I was Richard's sole case manager. It felt as if the three of us were together in this very difficult situation. And when Richard was dying, this doctor came and made his own private good-bye. He quietly and soundlessly just held Richard's foot. It meant a lot to me that he was invested enough to do that.

The palliative care team was incredibly helpful at the most difficult time. It amazes me that people choose to put themselves daily in the way of such suffering, and I will always be grateful for their deep compassion and understanding.

Six months after Richard's death, I wrote the hospital to advocate for some kind of extra support for other people dealing with similar circumstances. It's not just the disease that needs to be treated; the whole person and the whole family need help knowing how they are to live in the world. There wasn't even a support group at the hospital. I believe that psychological support should be standard care for patients having drastic facial surgery and that the hospital has a responsibility to make sure patients get it. A gifted psychiatrist can form a connection with someone very quickly to help reduce the sense of isolation. Even a chance to talk openly while the patient is still postoperative would make a big difference, but the hospital was very resistant to these ideas. This was so sad because there's so much for hospitals to learn from asking patients and families about their experiences.

· · · · ·

Maggie noted, weeks after telling her story for this book, that "One of my children just had an appointment at the local children's hospital, and I saw a notice by the reception desk that said patient advocates were available if you needed help. In all the ten years of Richard being followed by his hospital, I never heard of such a person as a patient advocate or of anyone else who could facilitate solutions to some of the problems we were having with health care delivery."

His Name Means
"Rise above the Storm"

It was a dark and stormy night.

The weather system that started that February day in 2004 would eventually be called a weather bomb, and record books would be rewritten. In a twenty-four-hour period, this blizzard's devastating combination of 95.5 centimeters (37.6 inches) of snow and gale-force winds of 124 kilometers (77.5 miles) per hour created snowdrifts so deep and so high you could ski down them.

The province of Nova Scotia declared a state of emergency. It was as though everyone and everything was encased in a white cocoon. For most people, nothing moved for days. For a young couple and their young son, however, an extraordinary drama began to unfold at the height of the storm, after the power went out.

Kim was actually excited when she heard a storm was coming. She figured the snow would prevent her husband, Scott, from working his usual twelve-hour day as a contractor. Although they needed him to work to pay their debts, she thought it would be fun to have him home for the day and that he would enjoy playing with their son, Milo, who was almost two and loved snow. It was going to be a good day. She was cooking a nice ham dinner, and her favorite TV show, *ER*, was on that night. Kim smiled to herself.

Scott and Milo did have fun outside. Among other things, even though the truck was low on gas, they drove it back and forth, trying to beat down tracks to keep their driveway open. Scott figured he'd be getting lots of calls for additional work as soon as the snow stopped. Eventually, though, there was so much snow, the truck got stuck.

Around 6 p.m., Kim started to feel a bit "off." She was six months pregnant and thought the baby was giving her indigestion.

She and Scott had dinner and put Milo to bed. Outside, the storm intensified; inside, Kim's discomfort and Scott's concern also intensified. By midnight, when the power went out and they lost phone service, they knew they were in trouble. Kim was scared; Scott figured he had to get her to the hospital.

Scott started shoveling like a madman. All he had was a child's shovel, and it wasn't long enough to get under the truck. Scott, remarkably clever for his twenty-four years, rigged up a bar across the door to their house and winched the truck backward. Meanwhile, Kim was inside, lighting candles and trying to stay calm between contractions.

After three hours, Scott managed to get their truck to the top of their driveway. Only then did he and Kim wake up their son, dress him for the trip into the city, and put him in the truck. Disturbed from a deep sleep, Milo was disoriented and frightened. Kim's cries of pain, when she had contractions, frightened him even more.

Scott and Kim lived outside the city, near the famous Peggy's Cove Lighthouse. Under normal circumstances, the drive from their house to the city took about thirty-five minutes and was one of the most beautiful in the world, curving back and forth alongside the ocean's edge, past picturesque fishing harbors. The drive this night, though, would be completely different. All highways were officially closed. There was no visibility, and the snow was so deep that Scott knew he would have to drive fast to maintain enough momentum to get through the drifts. He knew he had to keep the truck moving because if the truck stopped, he would not be able to get it going again. But it wasn't fast driving on a twisting road during a raging blizzard that frightened Scott. It was the truck's gas light indicator being on that terrified him.

Miraculously, not only was Scott able to handle the truck on the unplowed roads and make it scale enormous drifts, he also found a gas station open that, although it had no staff present, still had power, meaning that its pumps were still working. Even more astounding to Scott, given the state of their finances, was that his credit card was accepted.

All during the terrifying and dangerous drive, Kim was in a state of disbelief that she could be in labor. She thought, *I'm only twenty-four weeks. It's too early.* Scott, on the other hand, had concluded and fully accepted that Kim was having a miscarriage, but he kept this thought to himself. He just focused on what he viewed as his job and only responsibility, which was getting Kim to the hospital. He didn't know it yet, but he'd find out that much more was in store for them both.

Kim, Scott, and Milo arrived at the hospital between 4 and 5 a.m. Kim was examined and rushed into a birthing room. Her contractions were close. Scott wanted to stay with her but first wanted to settle Milo back to sleep in his portable crib in the next room because Kim's cries kept waking him up. Then the hospital staff said Milo could stay only if he stayed in the same room with them.

Scott was incredulous. "The hospital was not busy, and I knew Milo would just go to sleep if he was given half a chance. There are times when policies should be lapsed. It was a miracle we had all arrived in one piece, and now I was being told I had to go back out in that storm and risk my life and Milo's all over again." Scott felt he had no choice but to gather Milo up and head back to his truck.

As luck would have it, Scott's younger brother had an apartment in the city six or seven blocks away, so Scott headed in that direction. He got as close as he could and had to leave the truck in the middle of a road. His brother's street, narrow and steep, was impassable. Scott and Milo were going to have to walk up the hill. The problem was that the snow was up to Scott's waist. He knew there was no way Milo could walk, yet Scott couldn't carry him and move himself, too. Scott grabbed a blanket from the truck, tied Milo in, and pulled the blanket behind him. Scott remembers: "My poor brother—he was woken at five in the morning as I handed him a screaming baby. My brother had been asleep for hours and had no idea what was going on outside."

Meanwhile, back at the hospital, while Scott was dealing with Milo, Kim was trying to communicate with a nurse. She recalls, "This nurse kept talking to me, rambling on with horrible statistics, telling me my baby was going to be born dead and that they were not going to resuscitate it. I started crying. I kept saying, 'I need a doctor. I need my husband.' The nurse countered with, 'A doctor isn't going to change anything. I'm telling you the truth.' I decided I just wasn't going to have this baby even though I was seven centimeters dilated. I remember wondering if she wasn't taking me seriously because I looked really young and had arrived wearing big boots, pajama bottoms, and a long shirt."

When Scott got back to the hospital, he realized that Kim was distraught and completely overwhelmed.

> I got hold of a doctor who spelled out the situation.
> He explained there was a 60 percent chance the baby
> would be stillborn, and I would have to decide whether
> the baby should be resuscitated. Then the doctor told
> me that even if the baby was successfully revived, there
> would be a significant risk of cerebral palsy and/or

blindness. I knew I didn't want that for our child.

The hardest thing for me was to be faced with these kinds of choices. Kim was beyond being able to make decisions. I knew I would have to do this alone. I felt I couldn't make the decision, and so I decided to let our baby decide. If he wanted to live, he would.

At 7:17 a.m., our son was born, and he let out a squawk right away. I was so relieved because the decision had been taken out of my hands. Because he was born at twenty-four weeks and five days and weighed only one pound, twelve ounces, we were told that there was only a slim chance he would survive more than a couple of hours or days. I thought, *Well, he's come this far. Let's see what he decides to do.*

Kim picked up the story. "When he was born, they laid him on my belly for the briefest second, and then we didn't see him again for several hours. The sight of him was scary. He looked like an alien. It was so hard to see a part of us in that state."

Scott jumped back in, saying, "We named him right away. We wanted to make sure that, if he lived, everyone would know who to root for. We picked the name Eli Storm because Eli means 'rise above' and, taken together, Eli Storm seemed to be strong. We thought he both deserved and needed a fighting name.

"Eli had to have heart surgery at two weeks of age. It was a frightening time for us. One thing that helped was a bulletin board they have in the unit with pictures of other babies who'd been there, and pictures of them now with little stories about them. These faces gave me hope that Eli could have a future."

Scott thought back to the four months that Eli was in the hospital and admitted that he was largely detached. "Because I had concluded, as we drove in to the hospital on the night of the storm, that Kim was having a miscarriage, it was hard for me to let myself fall in love with this little guy when he was born. Also, Eli didn't want to be held or cuddled, and so I pretty much stayed detached and went back to work. We already had huge debts and now had new expenses like gas and a car for Kim to get back and forth to the hospital. We were in desperate financial shape, and I had to work all the time. I couldn't visit except maybe one day a week. Working so hard, in part, was how I coped."

While Scott worked almost nonstop, Kim was going back and forth to visit Eli in the hospital. She explained:

> I knew I wanted to breast-feed Eli when he came home, whenever that would be, and so I pumped the whole time he was in the hospital. For the last month of the four months he was there, I was able to actually nurse him two to three times a day.
>
> I visited Eli every day. I almost always had to go alone. Scott was working all the time, and anyone else who might have been able to come with me had to stay at home and look after Milo. Milo wasn't particularly welcome in the NICU because he wanted to touch everything.
>
> But even though I went to the hospital every day, I wouldn't really do anything when I got there. Most days, I would just sit there. Often I would leave the blanket over Eli's incubator because it bothered me to look at him. He looked so weird. The few times family members came in to see him, I was almost embarrassed about how he looked.
>
> The nurses were wonderful. A number of them really bonded with Eli, and I was so grateful to them. Eli's

nurses always made daily and nightly entries about him in a handwritten journal they gave to me when we left the hospital. On Mother's Day, they gave me a series of framed Polaroid pictures they'd taken of him at different times. That was so sweet.

One nurse always came to me and touched my shoulder or my hand and asked me, "How are you doing today?" But I'm a very private person and I didn't really let anyone in. Some of the other mothers in the unit tried to get me to talk. I'd listen to them and I liked knowing that many of them were feeling the same way I was. But I didn't want to talk. I felt that if I talked or cried, everything I was trying to keep at arm's length would become real.

Kim and Scott recalled that they were excited to get Eli home, but things were still not easy, and they both admitted to continued feelings of detachment. Kim filled in some of the details:

Eli was on oxygen at home, which made him unhappy and interfered with his sleep. Scott was working non-stop and couldn't help much with the boys. Milo was potty-training and needed my attention, but Eli's care took so much time that I had little left over. Milo wanted to play outside, but I couldn't take Eli out. And I was unhappy, so my family and friends didn't particularly want to be around me. I felt very isolated.

I was depressed and kept trying to say to friends and family, and to both my doctor and Eli's doctor, that I was unhappy. But everyone had an excuse for how I was feeling. They'd say things like, "It's normal to feel a little down with all that you've been through," or they'd try to reassure me by saying, "You're going to be fine—just give it some time." I felt dismissed. No one took me seriously when I said I needed help. I started to think that how I was feeling was all in my head.

In hindsight, I realize I needed help even when Eli was still in the hospital. It would have been good to have had someone raise and address emotional issues with us. We were told where the social worker's office was located and that we could go talk to her, but we are private people and are not likely, on our own initiative, to go talk to a stranger. I wish she had approached us.

Kim and Scott both agreed that Eli's happiness and their happiness and attachment to him happened over time and in steps. Scott said, "Eli began to sleep better as soon as he came off oxygen. His sleeping well meant that we could sleep well. The next leap forward came when Eli started crawling. He was so delighted to be able move around and discover things. We have started to see him as a jovial person. He still doesn't love to cuddle or be held, but it's so much easier to relax and enjoy him as he has become more relaxed and able to enjoy life himself." Kim added, "I just had him at the doctor's for a checkup. He's doing really well on all the things they measure. He's big and healthy and happy. He has completely settled into our family and has become a best friend to his older brother."

Natural Allies:
Partnerships in Care

"Most of us feel better when we are seen and met with
authentic presence and regard, without condescension
or contrived intimacy. We feel good when we are treated
as capable, when we are related to as if we have the
capacity to actually undertake the hardest work in the
world, when a lot is being asked of us, but in ways that
build on our intrinsic capacities and intelligences."
—*Jon Kabat-Zinn*

"I need to be a collaborator in my care."
—*Kathleen Hipwell*

"The man who goes alone can start today; but he who
travels with another must wait until the other is ready."
—*Henry David Thoreau*

It has been said that true involvement of patients and families leads to better, safer, more compassionate clinical care and better clinical outcomes. Why then would anyone not want to deliver or receive care that is as collaborative as it can be?

In the complex world of health care, why would anyone want or think they could do any of it alone? Is not the provision of individualized information, support, and cooperation a two-way street? Are decisions about treatments and procedures made in partnership not better than those determined in isolation?

And, when patients and families offer their observations in a spirit of wanting to make things better for others, why would this ever be refused?

We Are Not Visitors in Her Life

Something's Wrong—Please Listen to Me!

That's What We're Here For

When the Brain Is Broken

It Takes a Team

Investing in Information

It Just Comes Naturally

Awash in Disappointment

Choosing a Doctor

Mama Carmela

We Are Not Visitors in Her Life

My mother was in the emergency department of a community hospital. She had broken her hip a month earlier and had been discharged. She was still somewhat disoriented, however, and we were concerned about possible cardiac complications. We wanted her admitted to the step-down unit.

My wife and I stayed with her for more than eight hours in emergency. A stream of staff, mostly kind and competent, provided care. My mother was unable to answer some of their questions, and so we supplied needed information and served as her advocates.

It was very fortunate that we were there for her encounter with the cardiologist. He came in and asked, "Who is your cardiologist?" We explained that my mother didn't have a cardiologist. He replied, with a tone of sarcasm, "Well, who put in her pacemaker in 1987 then?" We informed him that she didn't have a pacemaker and that perhaps he had the wrong patient. With no apology or explanation, he left to find the right patient. My mother would never have been able to sort through the confusion between the doctor's assumptions and her reality.

Eventually, my mother was transferred to the step-down unit. Two nurses—new faces—escorted us to the unit where another nurse greeted us. When we asked to stay with my mother as she was being settled in her room, we were told that we could not and were directed to the visitors' room down the hall. I replied, saying, "But we are not visitors in her life!"

My wife explained that she was a nurse, that my mother was easily confused in unfamiliar settings, and that we could help them settle her. She assured the nurses we would not get in their way. Other nurses came out of their patients' rooms, circling us as "the difficult family." Their reply was a firm "no!"

The door to my mother's room was shut and the blinds were lowered. When we were finally allowed to enter her room, we were told that we must be brief because visiting hours were over for the night. The nurse handed us a pamphlet stating that visiting hours would begin at 11 a.m. the next day.

We had prevented a potential error in the emergency room when a physician began to examine the wrong patient. Why couldn't these nurses see that we were important to my mother's sense of comfort and that we could help them assure the quality and safety of her care?

Something's Wrong—
Please Listen to Me!

I'm only twenty-four, but I figure I'm never going to have a horrible illness because I've done my suffering. Life cannot ever be as bad as it was two years ago.

As I look back, I'd say my problems began when I started junior high school. Up to that time, I had lived in a protected bubble at home. For example, for grades five and six, my parents paid me $300 a year if I didn't watch any TV. When I got to junior high, I realized there was a whole world I didn't know about, and I rebelled.

My rebellion manifested in a variety of forms. In grade seven, I became depressed and bulimic, and I started cutting myself. I'm really smart, but I only passed my year with Cs and Ds. My parents chose to take no action.

In grade eight, I got more depressed. I refused to go to school, complaining that I had headaches. I had a CT scan and was told there was nothing wrong with me. I failed my academic year but was put through anyway. Grade nine was the same story—I dropped out and failed.

In the fall of my grade ten year, a social worker came to our house. I wasn't going to school at all and, officially, I was considered "a truant." I remember sitting on the couch, talking to the social worker and starting to cry uncontrollably.

I was admitted to the child psychiatry unit. Clearly, I was depressed and pretty sick. Even though I was there for six weeks, no one caught on to the bulimia. They noticed only the cutting because I actually cut a vein. Before I was discharged, I signed a contract with my parents in which I agreed to take Prozac for three dollars a day. I was also supposed to go to a school for truant kids.

That school terrified me. The other kids were bad, violent, and into sex and drugs. I'd never even kissed anyone. I refused to do any work and stopped taking the Prozac. I became manic, and when I'm manic, I get violent. I was sent back to the psychiatric unit.

I was basically in and out of the hospital for the next two years. When I was seventeen and about to be discharged, it was determined that it wasn't safe for me to go home because I had threatened my parents. Instead, I was sent to a supervised home for adolescents. I hated it and refused to unpack. I stayed for only a day and a half and cried all the time. I was convinced that I didn't belong there and stomped back to the hospital with my bags.

I had exhausted my options. I still couldn't go home, and so, at age seventeen, I became the youngest person ever accepted into the apartment program of Metro Community Housing, which provides appropriate supports for people with intellectual/physical challenges to help them live independently. In my case, I was provided with an apartment, a case worker, and a social worker. I was also given financial support for living costs.

I was really excited about the idea of having my own apartment, but then I moved in. I quickly realized that I was a spoiled brat. I'd always had everything done for me, and I didn't know how to look after myself. I didn't know how to clean, how to manage money, or how to cook—I couldn't even fry an egg. I had an apartment, but—overnight—I was poor and I was completely alone. It was all quite a shock.

Eventually, I moved in with my best friend, who was also receiving disability assistance. We soon realized that what seemed like a great idea wasn't going to work, and our relationship began to unravel. I learned to love vacuuming because I could throw temper tantrums and say terrible things about her without her hearing. It wasn't the best situation, but we coped at a certain level for a while. And we drank a lot . . . a lot.

Time passed. There were good times and bad times. And then there were terrible, terrible times. Without question, 2003 was the worst year of my life.

For years, I'd been diagnosed as having "bipolar disorder NOS." This is a brain-chemical disorder and can be well managed with medication. At the start of 2003, I was on a medication that was enabling me to do well; I was starting to visit Laing House, a drop-in program for young people living with mental illness.

In January 2003, my psychiatrist made a decision that seemed to be out of the blue and without any logical basis, but with huge consequences. Even though this doctor had been treating me for two years and knew I was making progress, she decided that my diagnosis didn't fit and that most of my issues were caused because I was mostly "borderline."

At first, this notion of being "borderline" appealed to me because it meant that maybe I could get well by just changing the things I had difficulty with through therapy. Maybe I wouldn't need medication. Also, I presumed my doctor knew what she was doing. I quickly realized, though, that what she was really telling me with this new diagnosis was that I was completely responsible for my symptoms and that I was manipulative, dishonest, and overly dramatic to get attention.

My doctor decided to reduce my medication. I've been prescribed lots of medications over the years, and I've learned the hard way that it's not easy or simple to find a combination that works. Some medications have made me hallucinate or have given me slurred speech or twitches, or have affected my weight. I want to be well, but not with uncomfortable or unhealthy side effects. As my sense of myself started to change, I told my doctor that I was starting to feel really hyper and was having trouble sleeping. She didn't seem concerned.

I'm prone to becoming hypomanic, and I could feel this starting to happen. The sensations of being manic are fun, but I also fear them. I know that when I'm manic, I get violent and don't make appropriate decisions.

In June, while playing softball with my friends at the drop-in center, I was hit in the head by the ball. I had four fractures in the bones around my eye socket and developed a retinal hematoma. I didn't feel any pain because damage to a nerve left most of the left half of my face completely numb. Because I was also hypomanic by this time, I was amused by the whole thing. Standing there, feeling wonderful, and looking at my CT scan—which showed the bones that didn't meet and the giant protruding black blob of air that I'd blown into my eye socket by blowing my nose— was just so surreal. The ophthalmologist said I was the happiest patient he'd ever seen. The next sequence of events, inconsequential in isolation but deadly in combination, created a crisis.

I was supposed to have an early appointment with the eye doctor. I wasn't sleeping much anyway, but that night I made sure I didn't sleep because I was afraid of missing the early appointment. Because I didn't sleep, I didn't take the medications I usually take before I go to bed. To make matters worse, because of the injury, I had had to take some antibiotics for two weeks that had given me severe diarrhea and vomiting for thirteen days. This meant that any medication I was taking wasn't being kept down.

I'd been sick for thirteen days and knew I was in trouble. I tried to get admitted to the hospital because I could feel myself becoming out of control. I was told that I was okay.

Of course, I think I'm a genius when I'm manic. I'd been reading about string theory. I was convinced that I could fly and become pure energy and control the universe. Then I started hearing whispers. I tried again to get admitted to the hospital. This time, I licked the wall in the psychiatrist's office because I saw a dried drip mark on it, and I wanted to know what it tasted like. I was told to increase one of my other medications.

My friends couldn't believe that I hadn't been admitted, and they took me to McDonald's and laid down some rules. They told me I wasn't allowed to go out on the patio alone, I shouldn't talk to strangers, and I couldn't drink alone. While they were talking, I was hugging and kissing the table because I could feel its energy and knew it was so happy and wanted to be hugged. Clearly, I was losing the capacity to judge what was appropriate.

Things got worse. I knew I was getting too sick and thought, *I'll just end this now* because I knew if I were to get well, then I'd have to deal with all the embarrassing, stupid, and irresponsible things I'd done, including some promiscuous activity that had hurt my friends.

I got a pen and paper and was preparing to write a note, and then I was going to climb up on some scaffolding and jump off. One of my friends tried to stop me, and I started to beat her with the phone—I just wanted to knock her out and put her in the closet so I could carry on with my plan. It made complete sense to me at the time.

My friends and I went to the hospital once again. In the emergency department, I told the staff that I needed to be admitted, but the psychiatrist kept asking me to explain what was going on. I cried and screamed at him, saying, "I can't explain." And then I hit him. At some level, my mind was still functioning to preserve myself, and I was desperate to get admitted or arrested so I could be put in a place where I wouldn't hurt myself or anyone else. I figured hitting the doctor would do the trick. It did.

I was in the hospital that summer for three weeks and switched to a new drug. I kept trying to tell everyone, "But I did so well on the drug and the dosage I was on at the beginning of the year. Can't that be prescribed again?" Even though I was in the hospital for three weeks, I didn't feel leveled out when I was discharged.

In July, I told my doctor that I wasn't doing well and that I was feeling overstimulated. I'm hyperaware when I'm becoming ill, and I wanted to control myself. I was trying to be responsible and get help before things got out of control. The response, once again, was to up the dosage of one of my medications to level me out, but these gradual increases didn't work. I was eventually pre-scribed more than the maximum dosage for this medication, and I still wasn't leveling out.

I started to lose weight. My psychiatrist presumed the weight loss was me being bulimic again and that I was the cause of my own misfortune. She wouldn't believe me when I said I thought my medication was wrong. I asked to have a different doctor because I felt so insulted that this doctor wouldn't listen to me or give me credit for knowing myself.

My weight continued to drop. I tried to bolster my caloric intake, initially by eating healthy foods and then by eating cans and cans of icing. I eventually started drinking Ensure, but the pounds continued to fall off me. I could only fit into kids' clothing. I couldn't feel physical pain. I was so skinny and so weak that I had to drop out of school because I didn't have the strength to carry my knapsack or lift my feet high enough to get on the bus. I was so freezing cold all the time that I cried because being so cold actually hurt.

I was also totally confused. I remember getting lost at a local shopping center. Even though this place was very familiar to me, I couldn't figure out where I was.

By September, I weighed only 103 pounds. Given that my normal weight was in the 140-pound range, I had lost 40 pounds in four months. I actually thought I was dying of cancer. I was admitted to the hospital for two weeks and was seen by an endocrinologist. I had all sorts of tests, which revealed that the huge dosage of the medication that had been gradually increased beyond its maximum dosage had overstimulated my metabolism and caused a cryothermogenic effect.

My doctor wanted to reduce this medication very quickly. This worried me because my brain is very sensitive, and I knew if I came off this drug too quickly the effect would be to heighten all of my symptoms. I told her, "We need to do this my way, which is slowly." Her response was, "If you want to get better, you have to follow my instructions."

Suffice it to say, my doctor and I had very different views of the appropriate road to take to achieve my well-being. She finally got fed up with me and said, "We've outgrown our relationship." That's exactly what I'd been saying to her for the past few months. I was assigned to a new doctor, a specialist in mood disorders.

• • • • •

At this point, this young woman, who has been sharing her story with a sense of confidence, pauses. Her lips quiver and her eyes glisten with tears. She starts to cry and apologizes. She starts to speak again, wanting to explain.

• • • • •

This is so hard for me to talk about, but I want to tell you what happened.

At the end of December, there was a transition meeting with my case worker, my social worker, my new psychiatrist, and my old psychiatrist. I had thought long and hard about what I wanted to say. I turned to my old psychiatrist and asked, "You've had me as a patient for three years. I'd like to know what you've learned from me throughout the course of having me as a patient and how you will apply that knowledge in the future." Her response was, "I can't answer that."

After three years—after what I concluded were inappropriate medications and dosages and a completely wrong assessment of what my problem was, and after her thinking my weight loss was my fault—all she could say was, "I can't answer that!" I felt completely shafted. Can she really have learned nothing? Any answer would have been better than no answer. I still have no closure from this, and it really upsets me.

I am so grateful to have my new doctor. She accepts that I want to be treated as a partner in my care. She acknowledges that I'm my principal caregiver and that I'm smart enough and curious enough to figure things out. She understands that I want full clinical explanations, with proper terminology, and that I want to know about the possible side effects and interactions of medications. She is not threatened by the fact that I have my own Compendium of Pharmaceuticals and Specialties (CPS) and like looking things up. She appreciates that if I feel something is wrong, I'm usually right. She trusts that I will give her appropriate signals if I feel I'm not doing well.

I've learned so much in the past two years. I've especially learned that I need to be a collaborator in my care rather than merely a receiver of care.

Life is good now. I'm able to appreciate even the crummiest of days because there's always something wonderful to find in them.

• • • • •

Kathleen credits Laing House (www.lainghouse.org), the drop-in center, with her being alive. When her world was rudderless, it gave her a lifeline. "Kat" enjoys going to schools to talk to young men and women about her journey with mental illness. She is planning to go to college to study science.

That's What We're Here For

My husband is plagued by arthritis. He has had hip and knee replacements as well as operations on his back, his shoulder, and eight of his ten fingers. We are not strangers to the challenges of major surgery and rehabilitation. When Joe's second hip replacement was scheduled, however, we knew it would be different because we had moved to a tiny town in the country two hundred miles from the city.

Joe's surgery was going to be done in the city. I, however, was going to be solely responsible for his care at home, without all the postsurgical supports of the city. I was nervous about looking after Joe. He is a big man, and I wasn't sure I would be able to move him or physically support him.

Surgery was scheduled for a Monday, and we were told that Joe would likely be discharged on Thursday. I had three days to learn what I needed to know from the nurses. I felt that if I could practice each day, I could become more comfortable and confident about taking Joe home.

When Joe was taken down to his room after surgery, the nurses asked me to leave while they got him settled. I dutifully left the room. As soon as I reached the hallway, though, I turned around and went back. I explained, "I need to be here to learn what to do." The nurses said, "No, we'll do this. That's what we're here for."

The staff could have invited me to help. In fact, my husband, a very private person, would have been more comfortable with me helping him. The nurses could have included me from the beginning. They could have taught me a little bit every day, rather than waiting until the day of discharge to tell me everything I needed to know. It's hard to process all the information you're given just before you leave.

Talking while doing doesn't take any longer, and fortunately, a couple of nurses did talk me through what they were doing and what I would need to watch for. Even with them, though, it did not feel like a partnership.

When the Brain Is Broken

"When you break your leg, your brain sends you messages that you need to do something. When your brain is broken, though, those messages are scrambled or absent and you need others to be your surrogate brain. Give me a broken leg any day!"

And so began the interview with a mother of a young man in his mid-twenties who had recently experienced a second psychotic episode. She recalled events clearly, analyzed situations thoughtfully, and articulated her frustrations forcefully. This woman has been a public health nurse for years. If anyone understands health care, she does, but she is the first to admit that some things just don't make any sense.

> I knew Kevin was in trouble about a week before he was to fly home for Christmas. He had told us he hadn't been feeling well, was anxious, and hadn't been sleeping. I called a friend of his and made sure someone would take him to the airport. And then I found out what I needed to know and do. For example, I called his doctor, made an appointment for Kevin for Monday morning (he was coming home on a Friday night), and asked if I could start him on the medications he had been given when he had his first psychotic episode five years earlier. And because I like to have all my bases covered, I also found out what we would have to do and say if he was really in bad shape when he arrived.
>
> I knew right away. Kevin was escorted off the plane because he had become agitated when he tried to buy a beer during the flight and couldn't understand why the flight attendants couldn't process payment with a debit card. Then, walking down the bridge from the plane to

the airport, he stopped and took off his shoes, socks, and shirt, saying that he felt really hot. By the time Kevin reached us, he was in a wheelchair, being escorted by the police. He was unkempt, and his eyes didn't look right. I knew he was psychotic.

When Kevin saw us, he said, "I just need to get home. I'm okay." When we asked if he had brought any luggage, though, he didn't know. He swung back and forth between being rational and suspicious. I knew we couldn't take him home, and so I told the police, "I'm fearful. I know he is ill. He needs to be admitted to the hospital." The police called an ambulance.

The police then explained that if Kevin did not go voluntarily and safely by ambulance, they would need to apply a section of the Mental Health Act. This would mean they would arrest him and take him to the hospital for involuntary admission. I understood this and appreciated their caring, though difficult, description of how events might unfold.

While waiting, Kevin kept swinging in and out of control. He'd appear fine one minute and then be yelling the next. He tried to wander off, and security guards had to bring him back.

The journey to the hospital began with Kevin in the back of the ambulance and me in the front. My husband was driving our car to the hospital to meet us when we got there. Somewhere on the highway, Kevin tried to get out of the ambulance. The police were called. Kevin was arrested, put in handcuffs, and transferred to the police car to be taken to the hospital. As I moved to get into the police car, the police said I couldn't go with them. The ambulance driver piped in, saying that without a patient, he had no authority to take me. The police offered to call a taxi to take me back to the airport.

I felt as if I was in the middle of a Monty Python movie! I couldn't believe what was happening—it was night, it was dark, it was December, it was cold, my husband was halfway to the city in our car with my purse, I had no money for a taxi and no car at the airport, and our son was in a full-blown psychotic state with handcuffs around his wrists! I burst into tears, which was completely unlike me. Eventually, the ambulance driver figured out how to bend the rules to take me to the hospital.

At the hospital, Kevin was triaged right into psychiatry. I asked Kevin if he wanted me to be with him, and he said yes. He admitted to seeing things and hearing voices. The psychiatrist asked me if anything like this had happened before—*yes, five years ago*—what the previous diagnosis had been—*acute mania with psychosis*—and if he was on medication—*no, he had been taken off his antipsychotic medication by his psychiatrist three months after his first episode.* And then she asked Kevin if he had taken any drugs—*I smoked some dope*—if he was hearing voices or seeing things—*yes (as he was slowly trying to wipe something invisible to me off the walls)*—and if he was feeling violent—*no (but the psychiatrist had seen him earlier when Kevin had been much more agitated).* She finally concluded, "Yes, we need to give him some oral medication and admit him." You cannot imagine my relief.

Kevin was transferred to the mental health hospital and put in protective isolation. We went home at 2:30 in the wee hours of the morning. The very next day, we had our first taste of being cut out of the loop of information.

Overnight, we went from being the parents who'd been through this before, who'd been part of Kevin's recovery before, and who were able to provide background information relevant to the situation (such as triggers, details of the first admission, diagnosis, and what medication he'd been on after the first psychotic episode) to being parents who would be told nothing because the patient was an adult fully protected by the system's "protection of privacy." Even for simple questions such as "How did Kevin sleep last night?" all we'd get back was "You'll have to ask him; we cannot tell you."

Over time, I learned who might give me scraps of information and who would hold hard and fast to the privacy rules. Typically, it was nurses with more experience and a higher comfort level who showed some compassion toward us. It was still like a bit of a game, though. For example, rather than asking directly about how Kevin had slept, I had learned to carefully pick a "good" nurse and say, "Kevin says he slept well last night." And then I'd get back, "Well, we have a different definition of 'well' because he actually walked the halls all night."

As time progressed, Kevin was given passes to come home to stay with us on weekends. He was having his medications changed based on his symptoms and side effects, but we were never told what the medications were now. At the most, we might get something like "We've increased his meds because he's still showing symptoms."

We learned that if we weren't going to be given information, then we would at least provide the hospital staff with observations we had. For example, we might say, "Kevin had a good weekend, but he still doesn't seem to think this is a chronic condition that he'll have to manage for some time." We figured out that the more we talked to the nurses about things when there wasn't a crisis, the more they were willing to share with us. Sometimes I would find myself feeling clever when we'd get a scrap of information, and then I'd remind myself that this whole situation was ridiculous.

When Kevin was being discharged, I asked his psychiatrist, "Do you have a diagnosis?" He replied, "I can't share that with you without Kevin's permission." I tried to make sense of this: his brain is broken, yet he is the only one who can give the professionals permission to talk to us and provide information about his care? I wanted to scream!

Instead I said, "Okay—help me understand this. In the emergency room, it was important that I knew what his diagnosis had been from before and what medications he'd been on. And if I hadn't known, we would have all been flying blind because it took five days for his previous records to be faxed from three thousand miles away and they were illegible when they arrived anyway."

All the literature says (of course I'd been reading up on this) that the more stable, supportive, and enriching environment you can give someone who has had a psychotic episode, as well as the shorter the time a person is in psychosis, the better the recovery. Yet basic information was being withheld from us. What was I supposed to say if we had to take Kevin back to emergency one day? "Oh, I'm so sorry, we aren't allowed to know—you'll have to ask the person who is trying to wipe imaginary objects off the wall!"

We signed up for a nine-week course for families of youth with early psychosis, and this helped a lot. For starters, we discovered that everyone was similarly frustrated by the lack of sharing of information. It also opened up a lot of doors with Kevin. For example, we might say to him, "We heard last night that some families have worked out a relapse plan with their son or daughter." And he might reply, "Yeah—that has come up in my education sessions as well. I guess we should talk about it some time."

Weeks passed and Kevin improved. He was able to live with us and be supported during his recovery. Someone else in his situation, without a family with the means to provide love and financial support, would have been on the street, homeless.

We know that with each episode of psychosis, the person's recovery takes longer and is less complete. The idea, therefore, is to try to prevent reoccurrences. As Kevin's parents, we want to try to catch symptoms early and prevent another full-blown episode. I just wish we had more information to help us. We are relatively lucky—at least Kevin is open to telling us, when asked, about his medication dosages. His diagnosis? The "provisional" diagnosis remained: psychosis NOS (not otherwise specified). This is what the nurses told me I could say if required in the future.

If I had to rate the people we dealt with through all this on a scale of 10, 10 being the highest, I'd give 9.5 to the police; 9 to the ambulance staff; 8.5 to the emergency room staff; 9 to the psychiatrist we saw in emergency; somewhere between 7 and 8 for the nurses at the mental health hospital; only a 1 or 2 to the in-patient psychiatrist at that hospital; similarly, only a 1 or 2 to the discharge planning process; and a 7 or 8 to the outpatient services.

By comparison, I'd walk over broken glass for the psychiatrist we had in the remote community we'd lived in before, the first time Kevin got sick and his dad had to bring him home from college in France. That doctor's focus was community mental health. He knew we were there for Kevin and instrumental to his recovery. He told us everything and supported all of us through every step along the road of Kevin's recovery.

We move forward by inches. We watch everything for signs of relapse. We pick our words carefully before we say something because we want to keep the doors of communication and trust open with Kevin. Situations like this change everything about your life and your relationships.

There are gifts as well as pain. I feel I've become more empathetic. It has even changed how I read the newspaper. I now think that maybe some of the people who are reported as having done bad things are really people suffering from mental health problems.

It's so ironic that everyone talks about the importance of taking the secrecy and stigma out of mental illness, and yet our experience was that information was and still is hidden from us. Mental illness is treated differently from a privacy perspective. When my husband had knee surgery, the doctors and nurses told me everything without asking his permission. There's a double standard.

There needs to be a better balance between protection of an individual's privacy and involving the family so that they can provide the most informed support possible. The challenges we experienced in the name of "protection of privacy" need to be addressed and better handled. The overriding spirit and intention must be to provide the best possible care for someone. After all, we both want the same health outcome—a fully functioning member of our family and society.

At this point, this mother stops talking. She is obviously hesitating, thinking about what to say next. And then she lowers her voice and says, "I wasn't too sure about talking to you today. Then I asked myself if I wanted to be the kind of person I might otherwise criticize for not speaking out. There's so much to do about the stigma around mental health. But you know, I still wonder if I'll say anything in our Christmas letter this year about what happened to Kevin. I know if he'd broken his leg, I'd mention it. But to say he had a psychotic episode . . . I just don't know."

· · · · ·

At the time of writing, eleven months had passed since that frightening December. Kevin was doing well and living on his own and holding down a professional job that he loves.

It Takes a Team

Appearances can sometimes be deceiving. Picture a young couple, relaxing and playing with their healthy and happy four-month-old son before they have dinner. This delightful image, frozen as a single snapshot, shows neither the months of agony and panic that preceded this evening nor the many people who played important roles in getting to this moment in time. Where to begin?

"What was the most touching thing that happened to you when Jakob was born?" The dad doesn't hesitate and says, "The taxi driver!" His wife nods in agreement and tears spring to their eyes.

The dad explains. "It was two days after Jakob's birth and death. We were leaving the hospital and got in a taxi for the short ride home. I told the driver we had just lost our son, so would he mind turning down the music? We drove in silence. When we got home, my wife went inside right away. The taxi driver got out of his car, came up to me, put his hand on my shoulder, and said, 'We lost a daughter.' He was a complete stranger, but I'll never forget him. You might wonder what were the odds of us taking that taxi with that driver, but I find that every time we turn around, we hear about stillborn babies."

Shannon's pregnancy had been miserable: nausea beyond belief, continuous bleeding, and occasional high blood pressure. Regular testing, though, showed everything to be proceeding appropriately.

She picks up the story.

I went into labor at 6 a.m. on July 12, 2004. We called the hospital, and the folks there said to come in and be checked. When we arrived, we were admitted to the assessment unit, and a nurse named Judy was assigned to us. She checked for the baby's heartbeat but couldn't find it right away. She tried to reassure us by saying, "Oh, he's probably just moving around right now—I'll keep trying." She tried several times. We started to panic, and I broke down.

Judy took us into another room, where she told us they'd do an ultrasound. She began to gently prepare us by saying, "It will be good to check, but I think we would have found it by now." After the ultrasound, a doctor confirmed our worst fears and said, "Yup! He's gone." Apparently, this man is a genius and is the one called in for the most complicated obstetrical cases. He must see tragedy every day and has even lost a child of his own, but he seemed almost cavalier or nonchalant as he told us that our son, Jakob, was dead. Maybe that's how he copes.

Of course, my labor had to continue and play itself out. It took sixteen hours. My grief was like a drug. I felt like I was seeing and hearing everything under water.

The dad speaks again.

While Shannon was still in labor, a social worker came in. I hated her the first time I met her. She came in to offer support, but then asked about arrangements for the body and had me start to fill out paperwork for the death certificate. I almost yelled at her because I didn't want to see anyone, let alone talk about details of the death of our baby who hadn't even been born yet! Couldn't she have waited until the next day? Couldn't she have filled out the paperwork herself and just have me sign?

I have to say, I didn't ever want to see this woman again. She got a second chance, though, and ultimately, she was very helpful and an important support for us. After we went home, she stayed in touch with us by calling every week or two. She also recommended someone for me to talk to. And when we became pregnant with Noah, she helped us get used to visiting the hospital and becoming comfortable being there without freaking out.

The person the social worker suggested I talk to was the hospital chaplain, a priest. I thought this was an odd choice because I am not religious in any conventional way. I've never talked to a priest who hasn't tried to push something on me, but this man was a million times more a therapist than the therapist I ended up with. He was a decent and good person, and I appreciated his honesty. I remember asking him, "What do you tell people who ask, how can God do this?" He said, "I hope they don't ask."

Then Shannon pipes in.

Of course, we got to see Jakob that night, but not for long. But I do wish we could have seen him again, a second time, the next day. I also wish someone had suggested that we take a camera to the funeral home so that we could have had a picture of him there. The hospital gave us a beautiful memory box with Jakob's official certificates, a lock of his hair, a picture taken of him after I delivered him, his handprints and footprints, and the clothing he wore. We treasure this.

The nurse assigned to us when we arrived at the hospital that morning stayed with us long after her shift ended. She also came up to see us the next morning before her shift started. She stayed for half an hour. We talked and cried. I can't tell you one word that was said, but the fact that she took time out of her day to acknowledge our experience will stay with me as a warm memory forever.

The next morning, we were exhausted and in a daze. There were two nurses who were great with us. They seemed to be moving at a hyperefficient speed but were very kind. They urged Sean to get in bed with me and snuggle; we didn't know we could do that.

The dad now wants to make a point. "Nurses are fantastic. The way we see it, they do all the work. They bring you the ice chips, they rub your shoulders, and they're there for you as people. They treat you as the most important people in the world and form a relationship with you. Nurses seem willing to share themselves with you, whereas doctors don't."

His voice drops and his tone softens.

Time at home was hard. We had expected to come home with a baby, but our baby was dead. When a baby is stillborn, you don't even have memories. I remember that the night before he was born, I shone the flashlight at Shannon's stomach. Everywhere the light fell, Jakob would kick that spot. It was the only time I ever got to play with him.

When I went back to work, everyone asked how Shannon was doing, but nobody asked about me. Dads

get left out of the loop. In our society, guys are supposed
to be tough. I guess I was anything but tough because
seven months later, I crashed. I hadn't slept for a week;
I kept having the same images when I closed my eyes. I
was working as hard and as much as I could, but I kept
my door closed because I'd cry a lot. I'd never felt that
bad in my life, and I expected that I should have been
feeling better. After all, more than six months had passed
and, in theory, things were looking up. I liked my job,
we'd been on a vacation, and Shannon was pregnant
again. But I was in a constant state of panic and couldn't
handle anything.

I think the new pregnancy terrified me. It's not like
there was any point in time we could relax and feel confident. For example, if people have had a miscarriage at
ten weeks, then they feel somewhat confident that things
will be okay when the pregnancy reaches twelve or fourteen weeks. For us, our panic increased as time passed
because our worst point of reference was the last point of
reference.

Fortunately, ever since Jakob died, we'd been seeing
our family doctor once a week, just to talk. She could see
what was happening. She read me the riot act and said
I had to take time off of work. She wanted me to take
two months off—we compromised on one. She also gave
me some structure, some things I had to do: I had to eat
well, get daily exercise, and leave the house every day. I
spent a lot of time bawling in a park I found. I just let it
all hang out.

When asked what helped them with their grief and their fears around the second pregnancy, they answer together:

> A bunch of things, really. First of all, Noah was a very active baby and moved at thirteen weeks, so that helped. Also, the fact that we could see our family doctor every week and that everyone in her office was so welcoming and kind and understanding gave us regular support we cherished. We also rented a Doppler machine so we could test for the baby's heartbeat when we were stressing out. Our family doctor helped us not let this become an obsession and get out of control. She told us to use the machine only twice a day, and then only once a day, and then to go a couple of days without using it.
>
> We also hooked up with a website for people who had lost a child. It was comforting to not have to explain ourselves to any of these people. They knew. We knew. And they had tips and coping strategies that were so helpful to us. We could even offer advice to others based on our experiences.

Shannon provides more details about the support they received.

> I was able to connect with a couple of mothers locally who had had a stillborn child. Sometimes I just needed to talk to someone who would listen and who understood what I was talking about. Another woman I knew from work had a child who died when she was five years old. This woman sent me a Mother's Day card that May. She understood that we were still mothers.

During the second pregnancy, we had fabulous attention and care. We had ultrasounds once a month and were checked once a week for planning scores. We were given every assessment and indication possible that this baby seemed lively and fine. As we got closer to the end of the pregnancy, however, we became terrified. At thirty-seven weeks, we'd had it. We couldn't stand the stress and asked to be induced. We were prepared with a speech about how we wouldn't leave the doctor's office, but we didn't have to give the speech. The doctor understood what we were going through. He said he'd do a test to make sure the baby's lungs were mature and, if so, we'd be good to go!

I was induced at thirty-seven weeks. The contractions were four minutes apart and the labor went on, seemingly forever. After twenty-nine hours, the fetal heart rate dropped from 160 to 80. Within thirty seconds, we went from having just a single nurse in our room to having a doctor, a resident, some medical students, and several nurses. The intensity was palpable as I was told, "This baby is going to be born in the next five minutes or we're going to do a cesarean section." You cannot imagine our fear.

Within five minutes, Noah was born, and he cried right away. Our family doctor had tears pouring down her face. In fact, I think everyone in the room was crying. Finally, we experienced pure joy after a day full of panic.

When you come home with a new baby, you suddenly think, *What do I do with him?* We now have a new person to add to our list of heroes! The public health nurse has saved our sanity more than once. She helped me through my breasts becoming engorged; she determined that Noah had a hernia and needed surgery (successful); she just drops in to say hi; and she recommended a nearby family resource center. We go to the family resource center regularly, and there's another public health nurse who comes to that center every Wednesday. I always know there's someone I can easily check in with for reassurance.

Amid all these shared memories, Sean and Shannon hardly ever take their eyes off Noah. These three are each delightful and are clearly delighting in one another. They are, however, the first to say they didn't get to this point in time alone. They give testimony to the fact that it takes a team to support grief, to nurture a pregnancy, and to reinforce the early days, weeks, and months of becoming a family.

Investing in Information

The recovery room nurses always told me that my maxillofacial surgery patients were easy to manage postoperatively. They said they could tell that my patients were well prepared. I appreciated their positive comments. I don't mean to sound like I'm blowing my own horn, but recovery room nurses know their stuff. They can even tell you what level of anxiety a patient had been feeling when being anesthetized.

I knew a nurse who had jaw reconstruction and who understood what it was like to have her jaw wired closed. I would always try to get her to talk to my patients before they went in for surgery. I would also tell my patients, when they were coming to see me, to write down their questions. I told them, "You might be nervous and forget to ask me what's on your mind."

And in the evenings, I would call every patient I'd operated on that day to see how they were doing. These calls tended to confirm my hunch that people are usually uptight when they're coming in for surgery, even if it's only day surgery, and they aren't always paying attention, even to written postoperative instructions.

I started making these calls for a selfish reason: I was practicing by myself and I didn't particularly want to get called at midnight. Adding an hour of phone calls to the end of my workday gave me my nights and addressed patients' concerns before they became serious problems.

All the problems I'd seen in my years of becoming a surgeon boiled down to communication issues. I just talked to my patients the way I'd like someone to talk to me.

It Just Comes Naturally

Dr. Ann-Marie Thomas is Director of Inpatient Physical Medicine and Rehabilitation Services and Medical Director of Neuromuscular Rehabilitation at Spaulding Rehabilitation Hospital. She is also an instructor at Harvard Medical School. In 2001, Dr. Thomas was given the Compassionate Caregiver Award by the Kenneth B. Schwartz Center.

When asked what it felt like to be singled out for the Compassionate Caregiver Award, Dr. Ann-Marie Thomas said, "The hardest part about getting this award is that what I consider everyday care is what others think makes me stand out. I don't think what I do is special."

When pressed, Dr. Thomas admits that she can see some differences between the way she practices medicine and what others do. She quickly adds that she would prefer not to stand out, that she would prefer others do what she does. Dr. Thomas believes that the way she practices medicine is simply common sense. She adds, "It also gets the best results for my patients."

Dr. Thomas elaborates on four elements of her approach, which she says "just comes naturally":

I actually spend enough time with patients to get to know them. Nobody is just their medical problem. When somebody presents with a sore shoulder, I need to find out about that patient's whole life. I've found that the more you invest in the relationship with a patient, the more you'll get back. They open up and tell you everything. I learn things that affect my decisions about treatment and care.

I'm stunned that doctors can see patients so quickly. They just fly in and out. When I went to see a doctor recently, I had my mouth open to ask a question, but he was already gone. I made another appointment, and when he came in, before he could open his mouth, I said, "I'm just here to talk."

My "patient" is both the patient *and* his or her extended family. This view is especially important in my world of rehabilitative medicine, where problems are often complicated, chronic or progressive, and emotionally challenging. I recall a particular patient who was a retired neurologist with a debilitating brain disorder. He had deteriorated to the point where he could no longer be managed at home. I spent a huge amount of time with this man's wife, helping her contact and consult with family, listening to her host of worries, and comforting her through the decisions she had to make. When she first approached me, it was a busy day, and so I suggested, "I have only five minutes right now, but let's use our time together to figure out when we can get together for half an hour." I put her on my schedule later that day.

I'm a big advocate for having an educated patient, and, if the patient can't learn, then I make sure I educate someone else in the family. I want my patients to become partners in their care. To do that, they have to know everything—what they have, what's being done, why it's being done, what their medications are, what side effects to watch for, and what to expect and ask for when they go to see other doctors. The returns on this are huge. Patients are more compliant with their medications and treatments. If I'm away, even though I leave complete and exhaustive notes, the patient helps educate the doctor filling in for me.

It is important to empower people at the beginning of the relationship. I give patients and families my email address so they can send me their questions and concerns. They also know they can call me if they are in a bind.

My work often combines elements of physical rehabilitation with addictions counseling. I recall one man who came to us because he had to have a limb amputated and because of his forty-five-year-long alcohol addiction. This man had been in hundreds of detox programs before he came to us, but none had worked for him. We were going to have to manage his withdrawal from alcohol postoperatively.

I got to know this man very well. I found out he had twelve children, all of whom had cut him off because of his alcoholism. I came to understand how desperately he wanted to reconnect with his family. I committed to work with him. Even when he was discharged, I would call him at home just to check in. If he missed an appointment, I'd call to ask if something was wrong. And he called me, not only when he was troubled, fearing a relapse, but also when he was overjoyed, having been invited to a family function.

Because I had also coached him on what to look for and what to ask for if he had to go to a doctor in his community, one day he called me from the emergency room. He knew something was wrong, but the hospital wanted to send him home. He was trying to advocate for himself but needed help. I spoke to the doctors and told them what tests he needed. The tests showed that he had clots in his leg and lung. Had he gone home, he could well have been dead in an hour.

· · · · ·

This patient wrote about Dr. Thomas. "There was something missing (in the detox programs I'd been in). I don't know what it was. Dr. Thomas took me—a weak, trembling, confused, and very fearful individual—out of a wheelchair and gave me the gift of inspiration. She talked to me whenever and for whatever time I needed, busy as she was! She listened and helped me understand the disease of addiction. She is reassuring and compassionate and has exceeded any medical treatment and attention I have ever experienced in my seventy-two years."

. . . . .

I take time to listen. I always try to be patient and to imagine being in my patients' shoes. Another example illustrates what I mean by this. I had a patient who, until she became incapacitated by ALS, also known as Lou Gehrig's disease, had been a computer programmer for the Pentagon. Her mind was completely intact, but she had lost her ability to speak. She was still able to communicate, though, with a keyboard and on the computer.

Many staff would not take the time to "listen" while she painstakingly tried to say what was on her mind. One day, the nurses were trying to wash her, and she kept saying "no." The staff were horrified and complained to me that she didn't care about being cleaned. Of course, I asked her what had happened. It turned out that she was saying "no" because she desperately needed suctioning. The staff hadn't taken the time to figure out that she was making an appropriate choice between her priority of being able to breathe and their priority of her being clean.

I told the nurses that "not communicating is not an option. We have to own this problem and figure it out." Working with the patient, we ended up coming up with a list of common requests she might have and creating a communication board for the nurses. Now, this woman doesn't have to take a long time to communicate her basic wishes. Now, it's simple and quick. All she has to do is point her head to a spot on the list. At first the nurses were resistant to working with this woman, but now they are seeing the benefits of solving the problem. The patient has taken time to praise them for their efforts.

It takes time to work with staff and to sensitize them to patients' points of view, but the returns are so easy to see. For example, some medical students and interns were just barging into patients' rooms as though the rooms were extensions of the hallway. I explained that the patients' rooms are, in fact, like their homes while they are with us. "Would you barge into someone's house without knocking?" I asked. That's all it took. Now they knock.

I love working with medical students. I just hope that what they learn with me sticks. I want them to know that I continue to be amazed by the power of the patient-caregiver relationship. I want them to know that I have learned that a big hug can be as therapeutic as an antibiotic, a smile as comforting as an analgesic, and a kind word or hand on the shoulder more uplifting than any medical procedure.

It's about being human. As doctors, we should not be on any pedestal—we should be partners in an equal relationship. I hope my passion for my work and for the patients and families I serve is contagious.

My ten-year-old says he was born to be a football player. Well, I was born to be a doctor. I wanted to be a doctor from the time I was four and was playing doctor with dolls and delivering their babies long before I actually knew where they came from. My parents tried to discourage me. I even tried to discourage myself when I found out how long it would take to become a doctor, but being a doctor is all I've ever wanted to be. Taking care of someone's health is more of a privilege than anything else I can think of. It's almost sacred.

Awash in Disappointment

The following letter was written by a mother, Donna, in the middle of a Sunday night, after more than two weeks of waiting and watching. The letter was a plea to a doctor her daughter, Jane, had seen a year earlier. The mother wrote to this particular doctor because he was familiar with her daughter, the cystic fibrosis team, and the team system. Perhaps even more importantly, this doctor was someone the family felt had liked and admired their daughter's determination to recover from an infection in her blood that he'd never seen anyone recover from before. This doctor had said that it had been "a privilege to be part of the miracle of her recovery" the year before.

At the time of the writing of this letter, Donna's daughter, Jane, was in her mid-twenties. Jane had been diagnosed with cystic fibrosis at four months of age. Donna's older son had also had cystic fibrosis and had died five and a half years earlier.

Dear Doctor,
This is what I have watched over the last three weeks.

Wednesday, May 21

Jane arrives home from Circus School and goes directly to the freezer for ice. Okay—a rib issue—could it be another stress fracture—or maybe it's just a muscle. The ice was applied—the modest pain numbed—maybe it's a muscle. It's been more than a year and a half since the last stress fracture, and we know what happened after that . . . the DISASTROUS hospital stay. Let's hope it's just muscle.

Sunday, May 25

Jane is on the sofa and pale. Yes, it's the rib—full out and full pain. Okay, then off to bed for full rest—see if we can't rest this into relief from the pain. Try lots of ibuprofen for inflammation and pain relief. Just stay in bed to allow it to heal. Oh, and how about we do two extra masks and extra sessions of physio every day from now on. Let's keep this from getting out of hand.

Tuesday, May 27

No one has to be this miserable--let's get something for the pain. Total fatigue--touch of fever-pure exhaustion from fighting the pain. Oh, and a prescription for antibiotics, too. Let's be really safe and go back on those-after just three days, off of them. Coughing is hard with a sore rib. All the extra care we can have, that we need, so this doesn't get out of hand.

A call to the cystic fibrosis nurse coordinator for advice. The head doctor is out of town. A call to another doctor who prescribes Tylenol with codeine. I go to pick it up--oh, it's not there. Prescriptions like that need to be picked up at the doctor's office to take to the dispensary. We didn't know that. So off to the office and then back to the dispensary-paper in hand--to get the pills. Lucky I'd told Jane I'd go pick them up--she would have collapsed in pain with all the going back and forth.

Wednesday, May 28

Pain pills helped for sleeping and resting. With the rest and the physio and masks, maybe the cough will stay under control. Let's be patient and the healing should be starting.

Thursday, May 29

Out of bed and off to the airport at supper time to pick up Jane's friend from Boston. Taking it slowly--a nice distraction from the hard week of pain and fatigue.

Friday, May 30

A slow approach to the day-a walk in the park-and out for dinner. Pain can be lived with-but oh so tired. Tylenol with codeine will do that. But lots of masks and physio should help keep that cough from sneaking up.

Saturday, May 31

Sore, but not as bad-but so tired and short of breath . . . really short of breath. So short of breath that a walk up the stairs is trouble. One block up the street is trouble. Damn. It seems we're in trouble. Those extra masks are some relief. The physio should be helping. This is June-- asthma time of year--could it be that? The cough isn't that bad, but the shortness of breath-not good. Jane thinks prednisone should help. Let's just start with a few days at fifty milligrams and see. That should help ease the shortness of breath.

Sunday, June 1

A day of worry and wait. Maybe the breathing will be better tomorrow. Those extra masks, physio-not so much pain now. That rib must be healing. No fevers, not too full a chest-- it must be allergies. Surely, the prednisone will kick in and ease that shortness of breath.

Monday, June 2

Okay, we'll watch this puffing, shortness of breath, breathing coming and going--we should get something. This is hard to watch.

Tuesday, June 3

I can't take it anymore. I call the nurse coordinator myself. My thoughts--an IV solumedrol. They did that on one admission, and Jane thought it was the most effective treatment. Maybe we could try that? Could it be done as an outpatient? In emergency? Let's get some relief for this shortness of breath.

Wednesday, June 4

The nurse coordinator says, "Before we prescribe we want
to assess, so send Jane over for a pulmonary function test,
blood test, and an X-ray." Great! This is all done before
noon. We'll get some answers, some treatment, and some
relief from the shortness of breath and the cough that is
creeping up and getting a bit worse. The head doctor won't be
seeing Jane—but will let us know the course of action after
the results are in. Wonder if that solumedrol would just
ease the situation? Or do we need IV antibiotics now, too? No
calls by the end of the day . . . as we wait.

Thursday, June 5

Okay, it's 2:30 in the afternoon and no calls yet. What does
this mean? I'm calling to find out. Oh . . . the head doctor
won't be there all day but will call on Friday. Okay, we'll
sit here, waiting, watching Jane in her discomfort—short of
breath and with a cough that's getting worse. We'll do the
extra masks and physio, and we'll try to think that something
can be done here to keep us out of the hospital . . . because
we know where that went last time. But what has to be, has to
be. They'll be in at 8 a.m. and so we'll just wait.

Friday, June 6

Are those flushed cheeks from the high dosage of steroids?
Is that a slight fever? When will they call? What are we
doing here? It's Friday—it's too late to do anything.

   Okay, it's 2:30 in the afternoon—I'm calling again. I
ask the nurse coordinator, "What's up? What's the plan?" She
says, "Oh, we're just finishing clinic. We'll call you back
shortly."

   At 3:30, she calls. "Okay, the plan—home IV antibiotics
for two weeks. It's Friday, so we'll start it all on Monday.
Pic line in at noon, pick up meds in the afternoon. A run-
through with the home IV people. The X-rays don't look too

bad. If it were asthma, the steroids would have helped but haven't. Switch to medrol from prednisone."

What's that, I wonder, and why–and why not IV steroids? With all the planning for Monday, I forget to ask.

Saturday, June 7

Not such a great day--a bit achy, a hint of fever at the start of the day. But after all, we'll be on meds by Monday night. I see a thermometer on the counter. Has she been worrying about her fever? Is she not telling us, not wanting us to worry? It's a Saturday, so there's no point in talking about fevers. There's nothing that's going to be done until late Monday.

Sunday, June 8

It sure is hard to watch someone so short of breath. It sure is hard to hear someone cough that hard. It sure is hard not to be worried totally to a frazzle as you wait for it to be Monday. It sure is hard to have to be saying, "Sure, I think two weeks of home IV will do the job, dear."

The point is that <u>it is all hard</u>. So, here are my questions:

1. Why seven days–from Tuesday to Monday–before any single change to my daughter's treatment takes place?

2. Would it not have been appropriate for someone--a doctor--to actually see Jane? Or is she just the sum of her blood tests, X-rays, and pulmonary function tests?

3. Would a doctor, seeing her shortness of breath, not have recognized the need for relief for her?

4. Don't we all know that nothing happens on weekends? But illness and symptoms don't take weekends off.

5. Can you imagine the emotional toll here for our family,
   for these last days? Watching, rationalizing, worrying,
   quietly praying, pretending.

This has been long and rambling, I know.

What would I have wanted? That I call a doctor on a Tuesday
and someone sees my daughter, recognizes a situation, and
moves on it.

But what have I seen? That I call a doctor on Tuesday,
and it's now the middle of the night on Sunday, and we're no
further ahead. But how much ground did we lose while waiting?

The most important thought--<u>Where's the preventative
approach to cystic fibrosis treatment?</u>

For more than twenty years we have approached this disease
with "How do we prevent problems?" But for the past eight
years--and let's say it--under the umbrella of adult care--the
approach has been, "How do we treat problems?"

The distinction is crucial. A seven-day delay prevents
nothing. A seven-day delay provides lots of problems to treat.

How do we work to change this?

Can you and I have a chat to talk about it?

I ask this of you because of who and what you are and who you
have been for us.

Help us make this work better. We need to for Jane, and we
need to for all the others.

–Donna

· · · · ·

Five weeks later, on Tuesday, July 15, Jane died.

*Now, two and a half years later, Donna says that she is not awash
in bitterness that her two children had cystic fibrosis and have now
died. She says that she is awash in disappointment and frustration
that she hasn't been able to make the world of adult care better for
others with cystic fibrosis.*

Donna, along with her husband and her children, knew the world of cystic fibrosis and hospitals intimately. She explains that their experiences within the world of pediatrics had shown them all what the gold standard of care can be. In pediatrics, their experience was that the care of children with cystic fibrosis was focused on the potential for full lives, on problem prevention, and on involving and respecting patients and families. She even recalls, with some fondness, the day they learned that their son also had cystic fibrosis. She had called the doctor's office to find out if the results were in and was told that the doctor would call her right back. The next thing she knew was that the pediatrician was at the door of her house. He said, "I couldn't give you this news over the phone."

Both of Jane's parents had been very involved in local, national, and international organizations devoted to cystic fibrosis. In spite of their demonstrated deep commitment to the field and their intimate knowledge about the care of their children, Donna says that when her children moved from the world of pediatrics to the world of adult care, she felt she was labeled as aggressive, intrusive, overprotective, pampered, and spoiled. Donna asks:

Does expecting the best care for my children make me spoiled? Does knowing that a high standard of care existed one block away make me pampered? What is aggressive about asking for the same level of care in the world of adult medicine?

As a family, we had always put our thoughts together to see what we could be doing as a game plan, what we might want to talk over with the doctors, what questions we would have, what advice we were looking for. In the adult hospital, we never felt that the staff were partners with us. We felt we had to be the ones to know about treatment options and what needed to be done. We felt we had to know everything, to ask for everything, to start at the very beginning with every new person. They didn't seem to care, and they conveyed an attitude of, "Well, your child has cystic fibrosis—he or she is going to die."

The so-called "team" was fragmented, and they never pulled together. You never knew who you'd see because the doctors in the clinic and on the wards changed every month or two. The senior doctor, who was the one constant person, rarely came to see our children, even when they were admitted. If the person at the top of the chain isn't in the room checking on patients, what's a resident to do?

Very early on, in the adult hospital world, my husband and I asked for a meeting with one of the hospital vice presidents. We wanted to make a case for some of the difficulties we were having; to share some of what we'd learned from our children's years under pediatric care and also from our wide involvement in the world of cystic fibrosis organizations; and to offer our help to improve the situation, not only for our own children, but also generally. But all the vice president could talk about was "process" and "the system" and "the needs of the hospital." He had no concept of patient- or family-centered care.

I tried every avenue I could think of. I even went to the hospital's ombudsman. He listened with great empathy and admitted that he was powerless to bring about any change. I went through the social work department. I offered to help the cystic fibrosis nurse coordinator, explaining that my role was not to criticize but to be an advocate for the nurses and the important work they do. No one ever picked up on any offers of help.

No one can accuse me of having vested interests now, and I'd still like to help bring about changes to make the adult care of people with cystic fibrosis better. But I can't tell you how powerless I felt. I saw so many changes that were desperately needed, yet I was not able to make a difference. It is a source of deep despair for me.

Choosing a Doctor

I had just moved to another state to be closer to family, and I needed a new doctor. My daughter suggested the practice where she goes. I was encouraged when I talked with a helpful receptionist who assured me that some of the doctors were taking new patients.

When I went for my initial appointment, the staff at the front desk were welcoming and a lovely medical assistant took my history. I had all my records and paperwork from my previous doctor with me but especially mentioned that I had received two new knees in the last year.

When the doctor came in, she immediately sat down and looked at the computer. Rather than saying hello, she started grumbling at what she was seeing on the computer screen saying things like "This isn't right. Two new knees? That's bilateral TKR." She was criticizing what the medical assistant had written, which made me feel uncomfortable. She continued to focus on the computer, complaining and muttering, "We didn't take typing in medical school."

To try to lighten the mood, I said that I had all my records with me and that I had had a physical in May. She looked up and said, "Well you can't have a physical now. It's too soon, but they've booked you for a physical. I can't get paid for forty-five minutes, only twenty minutes!" All I could think was that her review and corrections of what the medical assistant had written seemed to be taking all of my allotted time!

The doctor seemed very frustrated and angry and finally said, "Well, it's not your fault, but this shouldn't have happened."

She finally faced me. I mentioned that I have both osteoporosis and osteopenia. She replied, "You can't have both!" I explained that I had different level ratings in my hip and in my back.

I also mentioned that I had pains in my legs and that I had read that this could be from a side effect of taking a statin, and so I had recently stopped taking it. She criticized me for doing this without having a blood test first. "I won't take someone off a drug if their blood levels haven't changed."

By then, I really just wanted to get out of there but asked if I could at least get a flu shot that day. She said yes and then stood up to leave. Her strident, parting words to me were "Now what you need to do is go to L.L. Bean and buy two down-to-the-ground down coats. It's cold here." I wish she had taken time to learn a little more about me; she would have known that I had lived in New England for many years, and, only in recent years, had lived in Washington, D.C.

I got dressed and into my car as fast as I could. The whole experience had been unpleasant and shocking and upsetting. I wouldn't go back there on a bet!

Mama Carmela

It was a gloomy morning in October of 2008 when I received a call at work from my eldest sister, Nena. I was surprised and nervous at the same time since she rarely called me at work. She was crying on the phone and I could not understand what she was trying to tell me. I asked her to please slow down and tell me what was wrong. She said she could not take it anymore and that she needed help. I asked, "What kind of help, tell me what you need?" She told me our mom, Carmelita, woke up with orange-size lumps on each side of her neck and was worried they were tumors. My heart stopped! I panicked, but hid it from my sister—I usually never let her see when I am scared. I was very scared. She said she needed help with finding a specialist to see what was wrong with our mom. I told her I would take care of it.

I didn't know where to start or what to do. I began asking friends of mine and some medical doctors I worked with for advice. After ten to fifteen phone calls, I finally found a specialist who took my mom's medical insurance. I felt hopeless and angry. I personally had one of the best medical insurances. My mom would not be seen by the best possible medical teams, because they wouldn't accept her insurance coverage.

The specialist I found was in West Los Angeles, but my mom lived in West Covina, at least forty-five miles away and a two-hour drive in L.A. traffic. Before we got out of the car on the day of her appointment, my mom looked scared as she held her neck, trying to hide the lumps. "Le duele mama?" I asked if it hurt. "Un poquito mijo". "A little", she said. It was a small comfort to me and helped me hide my own fear.

I held my mom's arm to steady her as we entered the building. It looked sterile and uninviting which only added to our anxiety and fear. My mom squeezed my arm tight, and I squeezed hers back; I didn't know who was comforting whom.

I checked my mom in with the receptionist who was eating a sandwich. She held her hand up and she finished chewing her food before she asked me to write my mom's name on a clipboard. My mom did not speak English, and the receptionist did not speak Spanish. Translating for my mom during her medical visits was pretty standard. I don't remember what the receptionist looked like or if she was rude or friendly. All I could remember was that she was eating a sandwich which smelled of onions.

Thirty minutes later the doctor peeked into the waiting area, called my mom's name, and then walked away. I took that to mean that he was now ready for her . . . for us. We walked into his office where a big wooden desk served as a wall between us. My mom sat down and I stood up beside her because there was only one chair. The doctor began asking my mom questions in English, and I quickly intervened, explaining I would interpret since my mother only spoke Spanish. He began to address all his questions to me, never looking at my mom again.

The doctor used medical terminology I did not understand, but I was afraid to ask for clarification. He asked my mom to sit on the exam table in English—maybe he did not hear me when I told him she only spoke Spanish. I walked my mom to the exam table and informed her that the doctor wanted her to take her blouse off. My mom and I looked at each other and, without saying a word, we understood each other's discomfort.

The doctor examined my mom without saying a word and after five minutes of heart and lung auscultations and palpating of her neck, he said, "Your mom has Sjögren's Syndrome." "Sjögren's what?" I asked. He handed me a brochure and walked out of the room, returning only to hand me a prescription. He said "This will take care of it," and left the room.

"Que dijo?" "What did he say?" my mom asked. I was trying to make sense of what had just happened. I was pretty used to doctors not giving my mom or us eye contact, not asking if we had questions, not treating us with respect, not speaking our language, not making us feel welcomed, not caring. But this was new. He did not explain what Sjögren's Syndrome was. What did it mean? Was it serious? Was it terminal? How did she get it? Was it contagious? Was the medicine expensive and would it be covered by her insurance? Was the medical visit over? Should my mom put her blouse back on?

We left the medical office with more questions than answers. I felt horrible but tried to hide it as I comforted my mom by telling her that we were going to get her medication and that she was going to get all better. Somehow I knew I was lying to my mom, but perhaps I was simply lying to myself.

Surprisingly my mom's lumps went away the very next day, filling her with happiness. However, this happiness was short lived. Over the next six months, she began to lose weight, feel tired and develop depression and anxiety. I decided to move in with her to help with her medical visits and her care. At age sixty-eight, I realized my mom had several specialists to treat her for multiple medical conditions that included her vision, arthritis, high blood pressure, anxiety, and loss of hearing as well as her regular doctor visits. She had six different medical offices all across Los Angeles.

None of them were welcoming, and none of them showed that they respected my mother or our family as decent human beings.

As a family, we decided to transfer my mom to Kaiser under their Senior Advantage Program for patients with the same kind of insurance my mother had. In spite of some horrible stories I had heard about Kaiser, I was pleasantly surprised how welcoming the staff were to my mom and our family. My mom had the option to choose all her providers and specialists who spoke Spanish, which made my mom very happy. I felt she had a team of doctors working together to help diagnose her new symptoms.

After numerous CT scans and biopsies, my mother was diagnosed with stage 4, peripheral T-cell lymphoma. My mom had cancer. After years of not knowing what was wrong with our mom, now we knew. We had a name. As bad as the news was, we were hopeful, and as a family, decided to fight this; my mom was ready to survive this "C" word!

I remember hearing from a friend that the medication my mom was given to treat Sjögren's Syndrome, an autoimmune disease that mainly attacks women, causes lymphoma in some patients. Why didn't that doctor tell us this before my mom took this medication? I should have asked more questions? Why didn't I ask? Why didn't he tell us?

At Kaiser, my mom was assigned to a great oncologist who spoke Spanish. He was a UCLA medical school graduate, and was young, kind, and gentle. He was also good looking and always smiled at my mom; he truly connected and empathized with her—my mom loved him. At times I was a little jealous, but the truth is, we all loved how he treated my mom and our family. The oncologist recommended that my mom begin chemo treatment right away. He went over all the risks, side effects, and possible outcomes with my mom and our family. He empowered my mom to make her own decisions about her treatment plan. I naturally began to ask follow-up questions, but my mom looked at me and said, "No mijo, dejame a mi." She wanted to ask her own questions. My mom was now taking control of her own medical care. I was very proud of her. I was very glad she had this great doctor.

Sadly, after 7 months of chemo treatment, my mom lost her battle with cancer. We lost her on May 3, 2010 at 2:15 p.m., a day before my birthday. She put up a good fight. I was so proud of her. I still am.

A couple of weeks before she passed, she asked to speak to all her children. When it was my turn, she hugged me tightly and said, "Te voy a extrañar mucho mijo!" I told her I would miss her even more. She gave me three pieces of advice:

1. Save your money.

2. Buy a house.

3. Go back to school.

I probably could still save more money and I still rent, but I did go back to school and recently got my Masters in Public Health. I now help give patients a voice to improve the quality of their medical care and their overall patient experience. I help patients have a better patient story.

Gracias Mamá.

· · · · ·

Armando Vallin's parents emigrated from Mexico in 1978 and worked hard all their lives. Armando, one of Mama Carmela's four children, had been a teacher when his mother became ill, but had always been interested in the world of medicine. His siblings didn't know what to do, and his father brought his mother flowers every day, but it fell to Armando to try to navigate the health system to get the best care possible for his mother.

Armando heard people's stories at an Institute for Patient- and Family-Centered Care Seminar in 2014 and was so inspired by those stories that he sat down one night and, with tears streaming down his face, wrote his own. This story is what Armando wrote that night.

Armando is now the Quality Improvement Coordinator at Petaluma Health Center in California.

More than Words:
Feeling Heard and Being Valued

"It is ironic that awareness, intentionality, and kindness
may still be sadly undernourished in many hospital
settings, especially since these qualities are what hospitals
are ostensibly all about. The very word 'hospital' betokens
'hospitality,' an honored greeting, a true receiving. But
somehow it is still all too easy within hospitals and the stream
of medical care, although nobody intends for it to happen, to
get lost, to not be met or heard or fully seen, and to not be
followed to the point of completion and personal satisfaction."
—*Jon Kabat-Zinn*

"To laugh often and much; to win the respect of intelligent
people and the affection of children . . . to leave the world
a better place . . . to know that even one life has breathed
easier because of you. This is to have succeeded."
—*Ralph Waldo Emerson*

What is the message contained in a greeting of genuine warmth? How important is a phone call to just "check in"? If I am referred to as my disease or symptom, do I disappear as a person? If someone asks about my life, apart from my illness, does that mean I am whole?

It is truly amazing what people remember from health care experiences. Although medical science can do so much to treat and heal people, it is often the human touches that matter so much and are remembered for years: being called by name, a gentle touch on a shoulder, the timely sharing of anxiously awaited information, the extra time taken for all the questions in the world, comparing pictures of children, discussing books read or movies seen.

A Triple Win

Surgical Suspense on Sundays

The Healing Effect of Listening

Tattoo It on Our Hearts

An Enormous Burden Is Lifted

Where's the Headache?

I'm the Full-Time Tenant of This Body

The Value of Asking Questions

I Didn't Feel Heard

A Triple Win

It was a crazy time. My mother was in one hospital, having had a stroke at age ninety-three. My niece was in another hospital, having given birth to premature twins. And my 101-year-old father-in-law was in a third hospital. Like a hamster on a wheel, I just kept going around in circles, visiting everyone.

And then came the day when it was decided that my niece and the twins would be discharged. In another hospital across the city, a similar decision was being reached about my mother. She was going to be discharged the very same day.

My only sister was an ocean and a continent away. It was up to me to get my mother and my niece and her twins settled into their homes. Everyone was anxious about going home, but no one was admitting it.

I got my niece and the babies settled in first and told them I'd be back. And then I took my mother to her home, a high-rise apartment building for seniors, where she proudly lived independently. I was afraid about leaving her alone—afraid she'd fall—but I had to keep moving.

I quickly went home to get something, and that was when I got a call saying my father-in-law had died. But I had to keep moving.

I made a phone call to check in on my niece. She said that the babies were sleeping and that she was okay. Then phone calls to tell relatives about my father-in-law and more phone calls to begin to plan a funeral. Finally, I called my mother, who replied, uncharacteristically, when I asked how she was doing, "Not too good, dear."

Shortly after this, a nurse from the unit my mother had been on called from the hospital just to see how Mum was doing. I think I burst into tears. I told her I was worried about Mum and also told her that my father-in-law had just died a couple of hours earlier.

Later that night, my mother's doctor called from the unit. He said, "I understand there's a lot going on in your life right now. You know, I've been thinking. We haven't actually completed the discharge papers for your mother, and so we think it's best if you just bring her back in. We'll take care of her at least until the funeral is over. We'll also do another assessment before we send her home again. We know that when someone has a stroke, we're dealing with the whole family." Amazing! He actually said that.

And so I took Mum back to the hospital. She was relieved because she really wasn't ready to be home. She stayed for another two weeks, and the investment of that extra time enabled her to live on her own for another four years. I'll never forget that doctor's compassion. His decision ended up being good for her, good for me, and good for the health care system.

Surgical Suspense on Sundays

My mother-in-law's health had been failing at home. She was admitted to the hospital to try to determine what was going on. After a week in the hospital, she was having trouble breathing. It was decided to do exploratory surgery. The situation seemed very serious, and the family was notified. My mother-in-law was given Last Rites on Sunday morning, and the operation was scheduled to start at 1 p.m.

The family was taken to a waiting room. Time passed. No one came out to tell us anything. By 6:30 p.m., I said that I would try to find out what was going on if we still hadn't heard anything by 7 p.m. I was able to wait only another fifteen minutes, though—I was desperate for some information.

My sister-in-law came with me. The first problem we had was that we couldn't find anyone to ask. There was no one to be found. We finally found a nurse who directed us to a phone with a direct line into the operating room suite. A man answered the phone, and we explained who we were looking for. He replied that there was no one in the operating room under that name. We were frantic. It was now 7:15 p.m. Where to turn next?

And then my sister-in-law remembered that she had been given a number to call for information. We found a pay phone and eventually reached the surgeon. He told us that the operation had ended at 3 p.m. and had been deemed a success.

Somewhat relieved, we were anxious to see her. Even that was not simple. After the operation, my mother-in-law had been moved to a different floor than the one she'd been on that morning. No one had told us that would happen.

Every time I think of this, my blood pressure goes up. We'd just been sitting there like good little soldiers, waiting. I wonder when it would have dawned on someone to come and tell us that she was alive!

◆ ◆ ◆

My teenage daughter had to have surgery on a Sunday morning. She had injured herself thirty-six hours earlier, and her knee was a mess. Waiting at home until the time for surgery arrived had been very stressful. My daughter had been in a lot of pain, and neither of us really knew how much damage had been done. Surgery would tell us that.

To some degree, I think we were both relieved when Sunday morning arrived. My daughter was exhausted from the pain, and I was exhausted from anxiety and from the surrogate pain of watching *her* pain.

I waited in a lounge on the same floor as the operating room. No one else was there. I didn't know what the surgeon would find when they opened up her knee. I had a book but couldn't concentrate enough to read. There was a jigsaw puzzle on the table, but I couldn't focus. I just shuffled through old magazines and checked my watch every ten minutes. An hour passed.

The next thing I remember is seeing a tall, slight woman, dressed in operating-room greens, coming through the door. She was smiling and exuded warmth as she held out her hand. "I'm the surgeon," she said, "and I'm pleased to report that the tissues around your daughter's knee were not torn—only seriously stretched. I was able to put everything back in place, and she's going to be right as rain in no time at all! You'll be able to see her in about an hour."

This surgeon put me completely at ease. Through her enthusiasm, she communicated that she cared about my daughter. And because she was so happy with the results, I relaxed into a smile.

The Healing Effect of Listening

I'd had this persistent shortness of breath that happened more and more frequently. So I went to my family doctor, and she ordered a consult with a lung specialist. I went to him and had all sorts of tests. Word came back that, thank god, my lungs were fine. Yay! "But why can't I breathe?" I asked my family doctor.

> DOCTOR (with a dull look and a shrug): "I'll send you to an ear-nose-throat specialist."
>
> ME: "Is there anything else that may be causing this? It'll take months to get that appointment, and I'd like some relief soon."
>
> DOCTOR: "Well, Dr. M. is a lung specialist, and he says there is nothing wrong with your lungs. He would know."
>
> ME: "Yes, and I am glad of that. But I can't breathe. Any ideas?"
>
> DOCTOR: Shrug . . . and more reading of Dr. M.'s notes.

Now, keep in mind, she had a patient sitting right in front of her—a patient who was telling her and showing her that she couldn't breathe well. The doctor never looked. She just read the notes from the specialist. *Ah,* I thought, *I guess the notes are more real than I am.*

Today, I had another appointment with a different specialist— a cardio guy. This had been set up months earlier because of a family history of cardio stuff. The difference was night and day.

> ME: "I know this isn't what you were consulted about, but I'm having this problem with breathing."
>
> CARDIOLOGIST: Making eye contact and moving closer and listening, "Tell me about it." He took a great history and did a great exam.

Now remember—he wasn't originally consulted for lung stuff, but he decided that the patient in front of him was more important than the note from the family doctor. Imagine!

CARDIOLOGIST: "I can't see anything wrong with your lungs, so we have to cast the net wider. Have you ever had XYZ tests?"

ME: "No."

CARDIOLOGIST: "Well, how about we see what they show? I am sorry I can't find why you can't breathe."

We shook hands and said goodbye. I walked away and felt 100 percent better for having been respected and listened to.

Imagine—listening to the patient has a healing effect! Making eye contact! Paying heed! Recognizing that just because one option hasn't borne fruit, the patient is the first voice one should listen to. It all seems like it should be so damned simple.

Tattoo It on Our Hearts

It was a holiday weekend. My son and daughter-in-law were frantic when they called to say that their twenty-seven-month-old son was "screaming all the time." I urged them to take Benjamin to a doctor. They went to five different providers that weekend, all of whom said they couldn't find anything. The parents kept saying that they'd never seen their son like this before, but the responses were all the same: "I'm the doctor, and there's nothing wrong with this child."

Finally, on Monday, my daughter-in-law Mary found a sixth doctor, who took an X-ray in his office. The X-ray identified an internal blockage (intussusception). He said that Benjamin needed to go to the hospital immediately.

At the time, I worked at a nearby hospital and so immediately went over to meet them. By the time the diagnosis came, my husband and son had arrived as well. The news was bad. Benjamin had cancer—a rhabdomyosarcoma of the bladder. This is a very aggressive tumor of soft tissue that was blocking his urethra and causing excruciatingly painful bladder spasms.

There were so many tests the first few days. Because Mary was pregnant, she couldn't be with Benjamin during the X-rays, and so Nathan, my son, went in with him. After the first MRI, Nathan came out sobbing. It turned out that the sight of Benjamin being anesthetized for this procedure was exactly like Nathan's freshly painful memories of putting his dog down three weeks earlier. He was not prepared for what he would see.

Benjamin was to have three weeks of chemotherapy to shrink the tumor, and then have surgery to remove his bladder and cancer cells in all the margins. He would be in the hospital for about three weeks. There was a time when he had eleven tubes coming out of his body.

We did not want Benjamin to ever be alone. He was just a little guy, and there were lots of new, painful, and scary things happening to him. Because Mary was eight months pregnant, Nathan didn't think she should be alone, either at the hospital or at home. My son also felt that Mary should never drive home alone. And so we developed a plan: Nathan and Mary would stay at the hospital with Benjamin, and when they couldn't stay, my husband and I would stay.

And then we found out that the hospital had an "only one parent overnight" rule. We got the "one parent" lecture, and I asked the head nurse for the rationale for this policy. She told us it was because of fire regulations, but I was able to find out no such regulations existed. In the end, they allowed us to stay, but we never felt welcome.

One night, my husband and I stayed to give Mary and Nathan a break. I remember it vividly. Benjamin had an IV pump that beeped a few minutes before the IV bag needed to be changed. If you waited until the last minute, you would get a very persistent and loud beep. I wanted to avoid that because Benjamin had had a difficult day and I didn't want him to waken. I called the nurse and quietly explained my request. She came in, with a heavy sigh, and fixed the IV. On her way out, she slammed the door, waking Benjamin. I was able to settle him, but I was so angry I was awake for hours. It was one of those little things I will never forget.

Did I do anything about it? No. We didn't want to rock the boat in any way because these people were going to save our grandson's life. We didn't want to make them angry.

Even though I held a senior position in nursing administration at another hospital, I always took my name tag off when I was visiting Benjamin. I wanted to be there as an ordinary grandmother, not as a nursing administrator. I felt intimidated in this new role on the receiving end of care. I found myself trying to be sure not to do anything wrong.

The problem was we didn't really know the rules. For example, Mary and Nathan, not wanting to leave the unit, usually ate in the hallway, outside Benjamin's room, at an unused table. Apparently, eating in the hallway broke some rule, but no one told us about it or told us what our alternative was. All we got were cold stares.

Family members of other patients were the ones who told us the most. They told us how things worked, who to avoid, what the rules were, and more. For example, in the intensive care unit family waiting area, there was a sign that said "Only two visitors at a time, and visiting only twenty minutes per hour." Other parents told us, "Oh, you don't need to worry about that. They don't really follow that. Just stay out of their way." Even though I'd been a nurse for years, I had never understood that family members know as much as they do.

I also learned that, typically, doctors and nurses have no idea what effect a disease like this has on a family at home. Mary and Nathan had to learn to manage complex procedures and equipment such as IVs and total parenteal nutrition (TPN) tubes. And then there was the sheer volume of medical supplies, equipment, and IV pumps that were needed on site for Benjamin's care. Even as a health care professional with years of experience, I was overwhelmed.

Layered on top of worrying about and caring for Benjamin, Nathan and Mary were burdened by financial pressures. Prior to Benjamin's getting sick, they both had two jobs to make ends meet. Just to manage the care regime, they had to give up their evening jobs and therefore lost income. They also had additional expenses for all the things they needed for home care. They finally moved in with us to have some hands-on help and general support.

The silver lining in this whole experience was how much I learned as a health care professional. I learned how to relate to families in ways that are genuinely helpful. I learned that the best professionals are those who are open to sharing what they know *and* what they don't. I learned about asking patients what was important to them rather than telling them what was important to me. And I learned that when people and families come to us, we cannot separate their physical bodies from their emotional and social worlds.

More than anything else, I learned that all of us who work in health care should recall the platinum rule, which says, "Do unto others as they want you to do." We should tattoo it on our hearts.

An Enormous Burden Is Lifted

I cannot adequately describe how I felt. I had just said good-bye to my daughter, Mary. She was taking the ferry to go to Vancouver and, from there, to catch the plane back to Toronto. I did not know if I would ever see her again.

By this point, Mary was terribly thin again and was becoming weaker every day. She had turned down an opportunity to enter the eating disorders program at Toronto General Hospital a couple of months earlier but now had decided to give it and herself a chance. I ached to go with her, but we both knew she had to do this on her own. This time it had to be for herself.

Our roller-coaster journey with anorexia was now in its second year. The ride started slowly at first and then gathered speed. Our family of four quickly realized that we were caught by a force over which we had no control. We all desperately tried to grasp for something to hold on to and things to blame. We searched for patterns, causes, cures, and hints of hope.

When Mary was first admitted to the pediatric hospital's program for children with eating disorders, we all hoped this would help. We were terribly worried, but also, in a sense, relieved. We had admitted that this problem was bigger than anything any of us, alone or together, could manage. One of the components of the program, like most eating-disorder programs, was family counseling.

Contrary to their intended effect, I can't state strongly enough how damaging these family counseling sessions were. Not only were they of no help to Mary, but the message communicated to the rest of us—me and her father and brother—was that we were all to blame "because these kinds of problems do not occur in a vacuum." This had the effect of digging the tunnel of my deepest fear—that something about my parenting had caused this horrible situation. My husband chose to deflect blame away from himself. He became more insistent and emboldened in his belief that Mary's problems were my fault because I had not made Mary eat breakfast every morning when she was eleven. And my son, angered that some stranger had implicated him as part of his beloved sister's problem, withdrew into himself, like a turtle protecting its soft inner core.

Mary was ultimately released from the hospital. She had gained enough weight but clearly had not gained the kind of understanding or peace of mind that would allow her to love herself enough to want to live. The roller-coaster ride continued. Mary had good days and bad days, my marriage fell apart, and my son managed to continue to achieve at school but became listless. My days were cloaked in a mantle of guilt, the weight of which left me with a feeling of powerlessness in terms of helping Mary or reaching out to my son.

I did read, however, and I talked to people. I learned enough about eating disorders to understand, at least intellectually, that watching Mary like a hawk and trying to have just the right kinds of food in the house would not really make any difference. I learned that some anorexics have to get to their lowest point possible before they can begin the road back. I learned that I had to let go of the situation, that even if I had been a cause, I could not be a cure.

For example, Mary said that she needed some time alone and wanted to visit a favorite older friend on Vancouver Island. I had to say yes. If I'd created this situation because of being overprotective, I now had to bend the other way. When I joined her several days later, I could see that Mary was getting worse. This was when she said she was ready to go into the program in Toronto.

And that was the day that I gently hugged her fragile body, told her I loved her, and waved good-bye as she headed for the ferry. She called me a couple of days later from Toronto saying she could get into the program in ten days, but she didn't know if she could last that long. She asked me to join her.

By the time Mary was admitted to the hospital, she was in terrible shape. Four days later, as I was helping support her in the bathroom, she collapsed in my arms. Her heart was failing her. She looked at me with terrified eyes and said, "Mom, please tell me stories." For the next three hours, I spoke without stopping.

I told her the stories of "Little Red Riding Hood" and "Three Billy Goats Gruff," two tales I had told her many times when she was little. Mostly, though, I told her family stories—going back to my grandparents, and how they ended up in Canada, and all the happenings in between, and how her dad and I got together, and what it was like the day she was born, and all sorts of remembrances of her when she was tiny.

As Mary fought for her life, I basically reconstructed her through narrative. I created a tapestry of her life by weaving colorful and comforting strands of stories. It was intense, and she held my hand in a vice grip while connected to tubes and monitors of all kinds. Eventually, after almost three hours, Mary's breathing changed. I raised my eyes in panic, silently asking the nurse, who had been present throughout, what was happening. She responded gently, "It's okay. She's sleeping now." And then I had the luxury of weeping.

A pivotal event for Mary had taken place. She had, in that moment of physiological crisis, chosen to live. She had hit bottom and had begun to return from her own place of darkness. It wasn't going to be an easy path, but she had clearly set her compass, her own true north. It was shortly after this that I managed to turn a corner myself, and I will never forget the moment it occurred.

Mary and I met with her new psychiatrist some days after her medical crisis had stabilized. Within the first five minutes with this doctor, forever to be a saint in my eyes, he made it clear that with eating disorders there was to be no blame; no one was responsible for this; guilt should not be part of anyone's vocabulary. The sensations I felt were profound, like the first sip of water must feel to one who has been lost in a desert for days on end, like the first flapping of a butterfly's wings when it has just emerged from a tightly wrapped cocoon, like the first glimmer of light a miner sees when rescued from a mine shaft of darkness.

This whole journey has been full of pain, worry, confusion, and fear. It did not need to have guilt added to the existing complexity of emotions. I try my best to be positive and to be thankful for the opportunities that have been provided for all of us to know ourselves better and to relate to one another with greater sensitivity and compassion. But it has been a long, bleak journey made more difficult by a professional who failed to understand that when a child is seriously ill, families are vulnerable and need support, not attacks, to triumph over adversity that tests everyone to the core.

Where's the Headache?

When I was alone at our cottage, I thought I was having a heart attack. I called 911. The paramedics determined that I was okay but told me to follow up with my family doctor.

I saw my family doctor two weeks later. I told him what had happened and also mentioned that I'd been having severe headaches. He took my blood pressure, told me it was very high, and said, "Go to the hospital right away."

I went to the emergency room. By the time I got there, my blood pressure had decreased a bit and so I wasn't considered critical. I was told to wait.

I waited because my doctor had told me to go to the hospital. I'm fifty, I'm overweight, and I'm a smoker. I know all that puts me at risk for trouble. I was scared.

I waited eleven hours and was eventually put in a little cubicle lined with curtains. And then I heard the doctor say, "Where's the headache?" I had been reduced to a symptom. I was no longer a person with a name.

When the doctor came in to see me, he let me know that he was annoyed with my doctor for sending me to the hospital. He said it had been a frivolous waste of resources. He made me feel like I was a hypochondriac, just wanting attention.

I wish he had called my doctor instead of yelling at me. I was just doing what I'd been told.

I'm the Full-Time Tenant of This Body

September 27, 2004. Simple enough. I was leaving work and heading to the parking lot to get my car. I was crossing a busy street. Halfway across, the light changed and I started running. And that's when I was hit. I'm told I flew ten to fifteen feet before I landed.

The ambulance took me to the emergency department. I was holding my arm and saying my leg hurt, too. They said that the X-rays showed a broken wrist and a crack in my leg. They thought the wrist might need surgery, but I was told that if I didn't put too much weight on my leg, it would probably heal. I was sent home with one crutch and an appointment to see an orthopedic surgeon two days later.

It was ultimately determined that I needed surgery on both my wrist and my knee. The crack in my leg was, in fact, right into the knee joint—a radial spiral fracture and a plateau fracture. Surgery was scheduled.

The operation took place in the afternoon. I woke up in the evening. I called the nurse because I was in a lot of pain and said, "My leg feels swollen." She said, "Of course, you've just had surgery." My leg kept getting more and more painful. I kept calling the nurses, and they kept saying, "You've just had an operation—this is normal." Around midnight, the nurses even convinced my wife to go home to get some sleep, saying, "The worst is over."

By 2 a.m., however, my foot was enormous and my leg felt like it was exploding, being crushed from the inside out. Now I had three nurses in my room looking very concerned. One of them was on a cell phone calling a doctor. They couldn't find a pulse in my foot.

It turned out that one of the screws that had been put into my knee had nicked an artery at the back of the knee and had been bleeding into my leg for hours. A surgical team was assembled. The pain was excruciating.

By 7 a.m., I was being rolled into the operating room again, this time to replace the screws, to repair the artery, and to make an incredibly long incision down my shin to relieve the pressure. Fortunately, someone made a judgment call not to send me for a preoperative angiogram. The surgeon later reflected, "If the bleeding had gone on any longer, we'd have lost your foot."

I was in the intensive care unit (ICU) for three days. I was still in a lot of pain. My wife Christy slept in the ICU. She would tell me every time six minutes passed so that I could push the button for pain medication. I felt like she was my lifeline. I can still remember the terrible moment when, just after Christy had gone to the hospital cafeteria to get some dinner, my nurse came to tell me that she was leaving to do a shift change. I felt totally abandoned and had a complete panic attack. I wouldn't have made it without my wife.

I remember the vascular surgeon visiting me and my alien leg every day. He had a grave, concerned look on his face. I tried to lighten him up. I wondered why this guy was so serious. It took awhile to dawn on me that the surgeon was serious because he didn't know if I'd still lose my foot.

As the vascular situation improved and people stopped worrying about any need to amputate, I began to experience a different kind of pain. As a result of the extraordinary swelling from the internal bleeding, it seems that the nerves in my leg had been crushed. What I was starting to feel was the knife-piercing sensations of nerve pain.

I'm the Full-Time Tenant of This Body

For two weeks this pain escalated to the point that the nerve medications could not be increased any further. Even with maximum medication, a person's breath on my foot was more than I could bear. Finally, the pain peaked and began to subside. Apparently, nerves—if they're going to regenerate—regrow at the rate of one millimeter a day. Given the distance between my knee and my foot, it will take two years to fully recover from this damage. I have another year to go.

After four weeks, I had more surgery to close the wounds and apply a skin graft. Finally, I was able to go home with a walker fitted with an armrest (because of my broken wrist).

There are a few things that stand out from my hospital stay:

- I remember calling the nurses one night with my call button. I had to call three times before anyone answered. They'd turned me off. You know, you can say you're busy, but don't turn me off. I've worked in customer service for too long to find this acceptable.

- Two nurses were great. One was friendly and would just stop in and take a bit of time to talk. She'd offer to get my wife juice. Another one, a career nurse from Oklahoma, also took time to talk and share a bit of herself. She'd also listen to what I had to say. Acknowledging me (and my wife) made the difference between a good nurse and a mediocre one.

- It was gratifying when people gave me credit for knowing things. After all, I am the full-time tenant of my body. I'm here all the time, not just for a ten-hour shift. I'm a relatively smart guy, and I was paying attention to what was happening to me. I was learning a lot. I remember knowing enough to stop a nurse once from drawing blood in an inappropriate position.

+ A positive attitude is so important. It's not always easy, and the days when I couldn't bring my mind up from the depths of despair were the hardest. Sometimes you need help to be positive because you're so exhausted.

+ Oddly enough, I was fond of my orthopedic surgeon. It's very challenging to juxtapose this with all that I've been through and what I still live with every day, but he has a nice, easygoing manner. He'd always tell me everything that he was doing. After things went wrong, he was very gracious and made sure I got the best care I could get in terms of vascular surgery, plastic surgery, infectious disease issues, and pain management. He was kind. He was always willing to listen to my concerns and put forth some effort to get what I needed.

While I was recuperating at home, I went to the burn clinic as an outpatient for graft therapy. On one of these visits, a nurse said, "I think this is looking a little red and warm." And so off I went to see the plastic surgeon, who poked at the skin graft. It exploded! So back I went to surgery to have my wound flushed and cleaned.

By the beginning of December, I was beginning to put a bit of weight on my leg. On Christmas Day, I threw down my crutches and joked, "It's a Christmas miracle." You know, if you don't laugh, you have to cry. The whole thing was so overwhelming and serious—I couldn't focus on that—making light of the situation helped me cope.

How am I now? My wrist is okay and I walk with a tiny limp. My leg is strong enough that I can run on a soft surface. I still have some weird nerve sensations. Will I have problems resulting from this in ten or twenty years? I don't know.

People tell me things such as "You're walking so much earlier than we thought," but I think it's not soon enough. Or they say, "You're making such good progress," but I think I shouldn't have to be going through this at all.

What will I tell my new little son about all this when he grows up? I'll tell him to look both ways before he crosses the street! I'll tell him to be careful out there! And maybe I'll tell him that my amazing scars are from a shark attack or a snowboarding accident when I was in the Alps!

· · · · ·

This young man chose not to sue for medical malpractice. He explained that he was already dealing with other legal issues regarding insurance and worker's compensation claims stemming from the accident. Additionally, as he says, "Although a mistake had been made, proving that it was malpractice would have been expensive, time consuming, and possibly futile. Also, the surgeon is a nice guy and I didn't feel compelled to attack him."

The Value of Asking Questions

In December 2002, my Christmas present to my eighty-year-old mother was an ambulance transport to move her to Massachusetts from a hospital in New York. It was a dramatic event, but I felt it was necessary to save her life. My parents had lived in New York their entire lives, and so this step was not taken lightly.

It's important to explain that my mom had a passion for learning. She was a bright, intelligent, analytical woman. She was a homemaker and community activist, offering advice and help to everyone. She had asked for a computer for her eightieth birthday. She used this tool to keep herself intellectually sharp and connected to her community.

That December, my mother had to go to the hospital for a surgical procedure. I was living in Massachusetts at the time but still managed to visit her every two or three days. The hospital staff would express their frustrations about my mother. They said that she had many questions about the side effects of the medications she was receiving and was asking about alternative therapies.

In my experience with older patients, health care providers are often not as respectful of a patient's and family's ability to ask questions. I even felt that my own engagement as a family-based advocate was not well received. I encouraged the staff to take my mother's concerns seriously, telling them that she was very observant and inquisitive by nature. In addition, I felt it was her right to expect respectful answers to her questions regarding her own treatment.

I am a physician myself, so I was in a difficult situation. On the one hand, as a son, I was experiencing the emotional ramifications of seeing my mother in distress. On the other hand, as a professional, I kept seeing the real potential for errors in medical judgment. In addition to my mother's questions, I would also ask questions, usually in response to an overt or impending mistake. For example, one night I saw that an error was about to occur with managing her fluid intake. Rather than challenging the physician directly, I asked questions and made a suggestion for a different approach. He commented that I knew "quite a bit about adult medicine for a pediatrician"!

On Christmas Eve, I noticed that my mother was extremely sedated. I asked what had happened. A nurse came up to me and whispered, "Please don't tell anyone I told you this because I could get into trouble. A consulting doctor has put your mother on Haldol." I couldn't believe what I was hearing. No one in the family was notified about this recommendation. My mother was too ill to give her consent. I knew that Haldol was one of the most powerful antipsychotic drugs and that it was inappropriate to use in a postsurgical, eighty-year-old woman whose agitation was caused solely by poorly controlled pain. That's when I booked the ambulance transport to bring her to our community in Massachusetts.

Once that crisis was behind us, and my mom and dad were settled into living in our home, I began to look for a primary care provider for my parents. I wanted to find someone who embraced the same values that I try to bring to my own pediatric medical practice—someone who believed in the family's right and privilege to contribute to their own care and care planning, and someone who viewed the family as a full partner in a two-way relationship.

It wasn't as easy as I would have liked it to be. We found many physicians who had no idea what it means to be family-centered and had no desire to learn. It took about a year, but we finally put together what we thought was a good team for my mother's health care. As it turned out, our expectations for my mother's primary care provider were not fulfilled.

Mom was diagnosed with ovarian cancer. As was her way, she had a lot of questions about the proposed treatments, their side effects, and whether there were any alternatives. The day before she was to start chemotherapy, she received a registered letter from her primary care doctor.

This was a registered letter—not a phone call. The letter said that the primary care physician was releasing my mother from his practice because she had been asking too many questions. He said, "The only people who stay in my care are those who do exactly what I tell them." He allowed no opportunity to question or attempt to reach a collaborative strategy. In fact, he felt threatened by the concept of a family–professional partnership.

As difficult as this challenge was to our family, imposed the day before a grueling course of chemotherapy was to begin, it motivated us to develop proactive strategies to deal with the limitations of a health care system that was not particularly sensitive to the intellectual or emotional needs of its consumers.

During my mother's chemotherapy, we were able to engage a new primary care provider. This physician embraced the concept of partnership. She celebrated my mother's cognitive abilities and affirmed her right to ask questions. This ultimately led to a collaboration invigorated by mutual respect. It led to the creation of a care plan that honored my mother's choices, dignity, and quality of life. It brought out family strengths that enabled us to endure very challenging times, including accepting a terminal diagnosis. Clearly, this physician understood that collaboratively planned treatment with dignity is more valuable than an autocratic approach to "cure." Cultivating a family's strengths is an ultimate goal of any effective family–professional partnership. We were blessed to have found a doctor who endorsed this philosophy.

•••••

Dr. Richard Antonelli is chief of the Division of Primary Care and director of the Department of General Pediatrics at the Connecticut Children's Medical Center at the University of Connecticut School of Medicine. He is committed to a process of care delivery called Medical Home. It has been endorsed by the American Academy of Pediatrics, the National Association of Pediatric Nurse Practitioners, and the American Academy of Family Physicians and strives to ensure that every child and youth, especially those with special health needs, receive health care that is family-centered, comprehensive, compassionate, continuous, coordinated, accessible, and culturally competent. In this model, the family is the acknowledged expert in the child's care.

Dr. Antonelli says, "This approach to care is what I try to put in place for my patients. It should be the norm in adult medicine as well." When asked how he came to this view as a doctor, he replied, "Respecting families as partners is fundamentally important. It starts in your heart. I can honestly say that families have been some of my most influential teachers in the twenty-five years that I have been in medicine." He goes on to say, "The health care system must exist to serve the needs of families, not the reverse. Families must be thought of as full partners in advising on matters of quality, compassion, and cultural effectiveness."

Dr. Antonelli's mother, Evelyn, died able to appreciate the value of having her story used to inspire other families to expect nothing less than full partnership with their health care providers.

I Didn't Feel Heard

At age twenty-four, I was diagnosed with adrenal insufficiency, which means that my adrenal glands do not work properly and therefore do not produce cortisol. Cortisol is a hormone that is necessary to survive. It is often called your stress hormone. Being deficient means my body can't respond to normal stressors such as being cold or warm, or excited, worried, or afraid. In addition, being sick is a major stressor on my body and so a common flu landed me in emergency.

The journey to my diagnosis exposed me to lots of doctor and hospital visits. Before being diagnosed, I initially presented with severe headaches. After a month, they became so piercing that I went to the hospital. My father had had a brain tumor three years earlier, which was initially missed. Of course, I didn't want to think the worst, but deep down I was worried and voiced my concern. The doctor initially dismissed my view and accused me of being a "drug seeker."

Three days later, on Christmas Eve, my family and I were told that I had a tumor in my pituitary gland and that it had ruptured. Steroids were prescribed which gave me a voracious appetite. This extreme appetite couldn't be satisfied. I recall eating a family-sized container of ice cream in one sitting, then feeling sick but yet somehow still hungry.

In mid-January, I moved to a new city and started a new job . . . and I ate. I couldn't get pants over my knees let alone my waist and so wore only skirts.

At this point, I was diagnosed with adrenal insufficiency and was started on cortisol and began to feel better. I felt as if I had started to get my life back. I lost the weight I had gained, and I recognized myself in the mirror. I took my condition seriously and learned as much as I could about it. I wanted to be healthy.

Flash forward to the day I ended up in the emergency department. The day had been exciting because I was out shopping for my first house. Halfway through a house showing, though, I looked at my friend and said I needed to go home immediately because I was going to be sick. Extreme nausea kept me in the bathroom for the next few hours.

I took extra cortisol but couldn't keep it down. I became very weak, both from being sick and from depleted levels of cortisol. I eventually called my younger sister to come and get me. I knew I needed to go to the hospital. I was so weak that I remember her bearing most of my weight as we went down the flight of stairs to the car. She drove up to the hospital, helped me inside, and then went to park the car.

I went to the triage desk and told them I was in an adrenal crisis as a result of the stomach flu. The nurse told me to stand behind the yellow line and wait. Knowing I no longer had enough strength to stand, I asked some kids in the waiting area to move so I could sit down. After a couple of minutes, I felt I was going to faint. A nurse I know walked by and so I grabbed her arm, explaining that I was in adrenal crisis and was going to faint and that I needed a cortisol IV immediately. She went to the triage desk, grabbed a wheelchair for me, and left me to be processed. At this point I became even more nauseous and told the triage nurse that I needed the bathroom immediately. Her response? "Just wait. This won't take long."

Thankfully, at just that moment, my sister came in. She took me seriously and pushed my wheelchair into the bathroom. She had to stay to help me because I could not manage on my own. I was now not only nauseous and weak but also in severe pain due to the adrenal crisis.

When we left the washroom, the ER staff took me immediately to a bed. I was thrilled—help was coming! A nurse came in and said she would start an IV to give me pain medication while I waited to see the doctor. I stopped her and begged her to understand that I needed cortisol and that would make the pain go away. I said, "Please don't waste time giving me pain medication. Just give me cortisol!" She didn't listen. After a handful of attempts to put in the IV, I had to interrupt to have my sister help me to the bathroom again.

As my sister and I were on our way back to the bed, I made eye contact with a physician I knew. I mouthed to him to please help me. He came in and I described my adrenal insufficiency and that I was in crisis. I explained that my endocrinologist stated that if this ever happened, I would need 100 mg of cortisol IV. With a very low blood pressure, the extreme pain, and my explanation, the physician agreed and gave the order.

As the IV started to give me the cortisol I so desperately needed, I immediately started to feel better. The nausea and pain alleviated within a short time. The physician came back to speak to me and asked if I wanted to be admitted or discharged. I told him to please send me home. I wanted to get away from the team of health care professionals who were not listening to me. I had suffered for several hours longer than I needed to.

As we waited for the nurses to do the discharge, I became frustrated again. The nurse came to give me a medication to take home for my nausea. She gave me a syringe filled with a liquid. It had a large-gauge blunt-tipped needle on it. Confused, I asked, "What am I supposed to do with this?" She told me to squirt it onto a spoon and take it orally. My sister, a nursing student, said "Are you sure that's correct?" The nurse responded "Yes, I just got this from pharmacy for you." I gave in. At this point I just wanted to get away from the confusion so I could rest, and so we left. I took the medication during the night as prescribed, but I still didn't think it was right.

Thankfully, I recovered very quickly and went back to work within a day or two. I followed up with the hospital's client representative, who worked with the team about the medication error. I was right: it wasn't the right administration of the medication, and I never should have been sent home with a blunt needle. The director apologized as did the manager.

The irony of this entire story is that my job, at the time, was in patient- and family-centered care, and I had worked with this particular emergency team in establishing a patient and family advisory council. I was known by the staff and physicians. Further, I am educated about my condition, confident enough to advocate for myself, and had a family member there to support me. Even with all of these things, I still wasn't listened to and I didn't feel safe. What would have happened to me if I hadn't had all of the "ins" and supports?

·····

The person who shared this story says she has forgiven and moved on from her bad experiences. She adds that she is even more motivated to help her organization really hear patients and families. She says, "I know that listening to the patient enables staff and physicians to be more informed and provide the care that individuals need."

Being Together: The Power of Family

"I am sure I only survived because of my doctor's
great care and my parents' great love."
—*Pamela Stein*

"Life loves to be taken by the lapel and
told: 'I'm with you kid. Let's go.' "
—*Maya Angelou*

"Few things in the world are more powerful than
a positive push. A smile. A word of optimism and
hope. A 'you can do it' when things are tough."
—*Richard M. De Vos*

When we're ill or injured, don't we all want our family and friends around us? It's family and friends who know us, who can speak for us if we have lost our voices, who know what calms us, who know what we can do, who will be there to help us in the long run. And stories from patients and families can help health care providers see what seed of hope or despair are planted.

Just as patients and families need support, so do health care professionals. Their close working relationships often create a sense of "family" at work. When these "families" are threatened, then staff need as much support as patients and families.

I Want My Children with Me

Smiles Tell the Story

Olivia's Story

It Was as Hard as It Gets: The Impact of a Global Crisis on Family-Centered Care

If Anyone Asks, You're Twelve-Year-Old Twins!

I Want My Children with Me

This Canadian mother was traveling with her four children on a ski vacation in the United States. Black ice led to a dreadful accident in which two of her children were killed instantly and one of the other two, her daughter, suffered a deep laceration on her face, along with a broken arm and a broken bone in her foot. The mother, with a broken sternum and humerus, was in excruciating pain. Somehow, in the chaos of the moment and in spite of the overwhelming nature of the tragedy and of her own pain, the mother remembers a great deal of the first minutes, hours, and days.

It was a sunny, winter day—not the kind of day you would expect an accident. But black ice knows no rules, and, as if controlled by an unseeing hand moving in slow motion, our car and a plow truck crashed into each other. Two cars, eight people; two dead, two injured, four emotionally traumatized.

Like a mother lioness, I fought to control what I could, fighting through the physical pain of a twice-broken arm and a smashed sternum and the emotional agony of knowing, instantly, that two of my four children lay dead in the surrounding bushes.

I held my youngest daughter, Chrissie, with my good arm and tried to assess her injuries. At the same time, I tried to calm my oldest son. Scott, a new, young driver, had been driving at the time of the accident and was terribly shaken and upset. He knew that Chrissie and I were injured and in pain and had already discovered that his two other siblings were in the surrounding brush, having been thrown from the car, dying on impact.

As my son gave voice to his own agony and guilt by saying, "Mom, I want to kill myself," I firmly replied, "Scott, I've just lost Nancy and Nate; I can't lose you, too." Little did I know I would be echoing this theme within the hour.

When the state troopers arrived, I asked them to speak to my son. I remember that the state troopers were so kind to take my distraught son aside to assure him that the accident had not been his fault, that it truly had been an accident. They made the same statement to the local media, all of which was ultimately a huge comfort to Scott.

At the scene of the accident, I made it very clear to the ambulance drivers that Chrissie and I should be taken to the same hospital. When I arrived at the hospital, however, Chrissie was not there. The emergency room staff were very accommodating and wheeled my stretcher to phones so that I could talk to my daughter's doctor at another hospital.

The doctor at the other hospital told me he wanted to operate on Chrissie right away, but I countered, saying that I wanted my daughter brought to the hospital where I was. The doctor retorted, "Well, you obviously don't understand. If your daughter is moved, I can't take any responsibility for what happens to her."

Speaking tersely, through teeth clenched from both pain and anger, I said, "In fact I do understand, doctor. I understand that I've just lost two of my children, and I want my others with me, here, now." And then I asked, "Doctor, are you telling me it's a matter of life and death as to whether my daughter can be moved?"

"No, just that I won't take any responsibility for anything happening to her if she is moved."

"That's fine, doctor—I'll take full responsibility!"

One of the paramedics, having overheard my side of the conversation, reassured me by saying, "Don't you worry ma'am! I'll go get her."

Meanwhile, the staff at my hospital were sensitive and caring enough to get Scott a stretcher so that he could lie down beside my stretcher and talk with me, eye to eye, quietly, privately. He asked, "Mum, are you going to be okay?" I answered, "If you mean am I going to die, then no, I'm not going to die. I'm badly injured, but I'm going to be okay."

I was so touched by the empathetic responses of the staff at this small city hospital. I knew that the nurses were upset because I could see their tears. I knew that the ambulance driver understood my anguish about being separated from my daughter because he had so quickly volunteered to pick her up from the other hospital. I could also see that the young doctor on call was gently crying, and I knew he understood because he had children the same ages as mine. I remember him saying, his eyes glistening, "I hate to ask you this, but could you please try not to cry. We're concerned your lung might collapse."

The hospital, with my permission, allowed the husband and wife who had been in the other vehicle—a plow truck—to see me while I was still in emergency. The woman was a nurse; she and her husband had children of their own. They were both overcome with the tragedy of the situation. Aware of their grief and sense of guilt, I tried to emotionally reach out to them and tell them that it hadn't been their fault. I think being able to see them was an important part of my own healing.

Eventually, Chrissie was brought to the hospital where Scott and I had been waiting for her. Surgery was scheduled right away for Chrissie, and the plastic surgeon explained everything to me. I was able to stay with her until she went to the operating room and was in a room across the hall when she came back from the operation.

While Chrissie was in surgery, I began to try to find out where Nancy and Nate were. Sadly, there was an atmosphere of secrecy, as apparently no one had the right to convey the truth. I pleaded with the nurses, saying, "I know they're dead. I just want to hold them one more time." It was only when the coroner arrived that I learned my children's bodies had been taken to the morgue, and I would not be able to see them. This was not the answer I wanted, but at least I had an answer.

Scott and I were taken upstairs to a big room with lots of bright windows. A phone was handy. No one ever raised the subject of money, of how much all this was going to cost, of whether I could pay.

A social worker called a priest and helped make all the arrangements for the air ambulance to take Chrissie and me home to Canada. She also helped find other people for me to talk with. Clearly, it was acknowledged that I wanted to try to remain in control, to continue to make all the decisions on my own. For example, I talked with the coroner about whether Nancy and Nate should be embalmed immediately in order to have a choice in terms of whether the family would want to have open caskets.

After Chrissie's surgery, she and I were able to spend the night together in the same room. The nurses cleverly put the two beds together in such a way that her good hand could reach out to hold my foot all through the night.

Within forty-eight hours, arrangements had been made to get everyone home to Canada. I recall that the air ambulance men were very kind and sensitive. They seemed to know how much every movement sent waves of intense pain through my body and tried to be as careful as possible. They also brought Chrissie a teddy bear to have and to hug. There were, however, some things they couldn't do.

For example, I had asked for enough pain medication to get me through the whole trip by air, including the time I would have to wait on the ground to clear customs and immigration in Canada. As it turned out, however, I was given only enough medication for the duration of the flight itself, and no one on the air ambulance had the authority to administer morphine. Tragically, literally adding insult to injury, my pain was allowed to get out of control unnecessarily.

At home, two hospitals had been alerted that a local woman and her daughter were being flown in from the United States. In spite of the forewarning, a communication breakdown occurred when I arrived at my hospital. Even though the hospital had actually assigned an inpatient private room for me, I was still taken to a cubicle in emergency and told to wait. To me, it seemed as if no one knew what was going on. After what seemed forever, someone came in and started asking a series of questions, such as "What is your full name?" and "What is your phone number?" Writhing in pain, I snapped, yelling, "I'm not supposed to be here. Call someone!"

Unlike the hospital, the local media knew exactly what they were waiting for, and they behaved like hungry piranhas. Scott and his father had to be taken through the airport via hidden entrances and exits to avoid the media mob. Relentlessly, the media finally tracked down Scott, calling him at home and hounding him with questions about what caused the accident and how he felt about it all. Privacy was not something the media respected. All they wanted was a story.

. . . . .

Eventually, the media went away, this mother's bones knitted together, her daughter's surgery to repair facial lacerations healed, and her son resumed driving. Emotional pain does not go away, however. Memories remain vivid, and included in those are the people who tried to soothe a family literally torn apart by a dreadful accident and the people whose actions poured unwanted salt into wrenching wounds.

Smiles Tell the Story

My soul was moved today. We have a husband and wife as patients in our intensive care unit who were in a terrible motor vehicle collision that killed a member of their family. They were both critically injured themselves, and both are on ventilators.

While I was making rounds this morning, I noted the incredible silence in the unit. I also noted that the nurses and respiratory therapist were gathered around a patient's bed.

As I drew closer, I saw that the staff had taken the husband off of his ventilator (bagging him instead) and pushed his bed next to his wife's bed so that they could touch each other for the first time since they came here ten days ago. Although they couldn't turn to look at each other, their smiles told their story of gratitude and love.

I am so proud to be part of a place that values kindness as an integral component of care.

Olivia's Story

A mother shares her concerns about her daughter's hospital stay through a letter to the hospital's administration.

Dear Sir,

When Olivia was born she was placed in my arms, and I was told, "You have a seven-pound, healthy baby girl." Five weeks later, I was trying to convince the doctor that there was something terribly wrong.

We learned that Olivia had a one-pound tumor in her abdomen that had to be removed. I had not even had a chance to be a good mother to her when I had to turn her over to strangers.

The surgery lasted about six hours, after which she was in the recovery room for several hours more. We did not get to see her in the recovery room. She was eventually transferred to the pediatric intensive care unit (PICU). We were permitted to see her at 5 p.m., the first time in ten hours.

At 5 the next morning, we called the unit to see how she was. We repeatedly got a busy signal, so we just drove to the hospital. When we arrived, we were told that the doctors were still doing rounds, and, therefore, we could not visit Olivia.

After rounds were over, I called the unit again to ask permission to visit and was told to wait "just a little longer." I waited and then called again and was told to wait another twenty minutes. I kept calling every twenty minutes, and each time I was put off. At one point, I was told they were doing some surgery and I would have to wait. They didn't know how long it would be.

I had been anxious up to that point, but then I got really frightened. I asked what the problem was, and all I

was told was that they were working on my baby and I should
call back later. It was now 2 p.m., and I hadn't seen my
baby for twenty hours! Not only was I frantic–I was also
getting very angry. Finally, I called again and simply said
I was coming in.

When I got inside the PICU, I found that the place where
Olivia's crib had been was empty. I panicked! Then I saw
her crib being rolled out the opposite end of the unit, and
I ran to it. The nurses were very lighthearted, saying,
"We're taking her to the floor. Isn't that great?" I saw
that someone had glued a pink bow to the top of my baby's
head, and I just lost it!

It's hard to describe what went through my mind at the
time. The nurses had no time for me to come in to visit
my baby because they were too busy with other critical
patients, but they had time to play with her hair and glue
a bow to her head. I wanted to scream, "I'm her mother! I
want to be the one to play with her, to put her first bow in
her hair. Who do you think you are, taking over my child as
though I'm unimportant and in the way?"

I was furious, and the nurses couldn't understand why
I was so angry. I wondered if any of them had children of
their own. I wondered if any of them knew what it feels
like to have your baby pulled from your arms and completely
controlled by strangers who sat at the end of a phone line
saying, "Just wait a little longer."

The last time I had seen Olivia, she had tubes
everywhere and was connected to a bank of machines,
including a ventilator. When did all this equipment come
off? Why wasn't I told that she was improving? I had made it
very clear that I wanted to know what was being done to my
child. I had called repeatedly. The nurses and doctors had
every opportunity to tell me what was happening to my baby,
even if they wouldn't let me in. Who do they think they are
that they can completely ignore the rights and concerns of

parents? Was there any need to continually prove to us they were in control, and we were not?

Later, Olivia was readmitted to the PICU, and we went through the same calling routine again. It seems senseless to me that only one nurse can decide if I can see my child, and, if so, when and for how long. No explanations, no logical reasoning–just "no"!

If there had been more information given to me that had made sense, I could have waited better. I know that nurses and doctors have to do their job, but part of their job is me. Babies don't come to hospitals alone. They have parents. I was only allowed to visit when I became irate, and so every time I went into the unit, I was irate. What way is that to establish rapport with a family?

I look forward to hearing from you.

> Sincerely,
> A Concerned Mother

. . . . .

In this hospital's case, the hospital administrator was stunned when she received this letter. In a very real sense, she was grateful that this mother took the time to write because she learned that practices on the floors were not as she thought they were. She used this mother's letter to improve care and change the way that staff worked with families. A clear commitment was made to family-centered care and to the education of all staff so that the situations described in the letter would never happen to another family.

It Was as Hard as It Gets:
The Impact of a Global Crisis
on Family-Centered Care

SARS. Severe Acute Respiratory Syndrome. Even today, the term provokes a profound response from those who were closest to the outbreak.

SARS is a severe type of pneumonia that is rapidly progressive and sometimes fatal. SARS is highly communicable and is spread by direct and droplet contact.

In the early months of 2003, SARS appeared as a new infectious disease. It originated in China and became a disease of global proportion in a relatively short period of time. International travel made it easy for the disease to move from country to country. Cases were reported in 29 countries, and there were 774 deaths worldwide.

On March 7, 2003, Toronto, Canada, had its first identified hospital case of SARS. By March 26, a provincial emergency was declared. On April 23, the World Health Organization issued a travel advisory (in effect for only six days). The provincial state of emergency continued until May 18. And then a second outbreak of SARS occurred on May 22, and the crisis didn't wane until August 2003.

During the acute phase of the outbreak, the Ontario Ministry of Health imposed strict guidelines with a single focus of wanting to protect patients, families, and staff. Many decisions, designed to provide safety for the greatest number of people, resulted in a terrible push-pull between the losses of some individual rights and the larger context of protecting the public good.

The severity of the guidelines varied from hospital to hospital, depending on the number of staff who had become sick with

SARS. Hospitals were rated according to a numerical scale. In hospitals where no staff had become sick with SARS, the rating was low and the guidelines were less restrictive than in hospitals where staff had become sick.

For example, in a hospital where no staff were sick with SARS, non-SARS patients could have one visitor. By comparison, non-SARS patients in hospitals where staff were sick with SARS were not allowed any visitors at all. Patients with SARS were not allowed any visitors, no matter what the hospital's rating. The different ratings and corresponding rules created confusion for the public.

Many hospital and health care professionals in Ontario hospitals were passionately committed to collaborating with and involving patients and families in care. They had worked long and hard to bring about positive changes in institutional and staff attitudes and practices and then suddenly found these gains compromised, overwhelmed, and paralyzed by forces beyond their control. Although controlling the outbreak and protecting people from harm were the objectives, there were significant consequences.

Overnight, hospitals and care practices went from being family-centered to system-centered. Overnight, hospitals went into what felt like a lockdown mentality: entry points were limited, all patients and staff were screened for symptoms, and security personnel made sure no one got past the front door. Overnight, many families were told they could not be with their loved ones. Overnight, the support, information, and additional care families typically provided were no longer easily available to staff, overruled by infection-control priorities. Overnight, all volunteers and several categories of staff, including psychologists and chaplains, were declared nonessential and were prevented from going to work. Overnight, health care professionals became bigger, taller, wider, and more removed from their patients because of protective clothing. Overnight, people became afraid.

In the world of pediatric medicine, it is common for parents to stay with a hospitalized child. During the SARS outbreak, however, if a child had been exposed to SARS, the child would typically be whisked away in an ambulance and that child's parents were not allowed to enter the hospital. If a child was hospitalized for a non-SARS reason but a parent had been exposed to SARS, the parents were denied access to the hospital. Nurses reported that they couldn't bear hearing children, from small babies to teenagers, crying because they wanted their mothers and fathers.

Staff would do their best to make up for parents' absence and facilitate some sort of communication between child and family. Staff would take pictures and send them home; they would ask for pictures of family members to be sent in. Cards would be mailed and emails would be sent. Phones became critically important to families trying to stay in touch and provide support for one another. Some calls would last for hours, with parents at home providing comfort for children undergoing procedures, and children being reassured that their family members at home or in other hospitals were still healthy and alive.

Hospital-wide precautions required children to be confined to their rooms. All playrooms were closed. In such conditions of isolation and boredom, children often became depressed and anxious. Child life specialists did their best to find ways for children to play and overcome this new profound sense of being cooped up.

Special toss- and target-style games were created; the closed-circuit television system was used for group games such as Bingo;

and one child life specialist even arranged for children to sit at the entrances to their rooms where they could at least see and interact with others and play verbal trivia games. Additionally, some of the volunteers no longer allowed access to the hospital made craft kits off-site to be delivered to isolated children to work on in their rooms.

Various stories from adult hospitals convey some of the tragic side effects of this outbreak. For example, a female patient in intensive care was unable to talk and was going blind. Her husband had been with her nonstop. Overnight, he was told he would no longer be allowed to visit his wife. Desperate to communicate, he emailed his wife daily love letters, which the staff would read to her and then laugh and cry together.

In one excruciating situation, all members of a single family had been exposed to and become sick with SARS. Tragically, they were all in different hospitals, sick themselves and worried about the others. Staff from these different hospitals did their best to be in touch with one another and to convey information and messages of hugs and comfort.

The mother of an eighteen-year-old boy who had been in a car accident begged to be able to stay with her son. He had been a bright, intelligent young man and had suffered a terrible head injury. He was just starting to communicate again. The mother was completely prepared to waive her rights to safety to be with her son and help him recover, but she was told she had no rights to waive. The system was larger than her love.

A calm, reasonable, rational, dignified immigrant woman, already struggling to adjust to a different culture and language, lost all composure when she was told and finally understood that she could not visit her sister. She was forcibly restrained by security staff until she could bottle up and contain her personal agony.

Hospital staff had to wear special clothing, including face shields and masks. Smiles designed to try to brighten a dark day were hidden from view. Patients could not even recognize a nurse they knew until that person spoke. Staff talked about how difficult it was to not be able to provide the comfort of touch to patients because there was always a protective layer of clothing in the way. Many reported feelings of guilt; because the striker suits were so hot, staff desperately wanted to just get out of their patients' rooms to be able to breathe again. Others described they felt "fog, fatigue, and exhaustion" from wearing masks for twelve hours.

Compassionate staff were caught in this web of complexity. They tried their best to keep patient and family lines of communication open and to show kindness in the midst of delivering care. And yet all the while, they were terribly aware that when patients are not surrounded by the support of family, their recovery is diminished.

Staff also talked about how hard it was to do their jobs while they were coping with their own stress. One woman said she felt like a leper whenever she left the hospital. Another was teaching a part-time course at the University of Toronto at the time, but when she arrived to give her class, she was asked to leave. Others spoke of being denied dental care for themselves or daycare services for their children.

And for those health care heroes who worked directly with patients who had SARS, they experienced "work quarantine." This meant they were confined to their wards in the hospital, no longer allowed to leave the floor to meet other colleagues for meals in the cafeteria or to go to meetings. And when these brave men and women went home at the end of an exhausting shift, they were quarantined within their houses and from their families. They could not leave their homes to do errands, and, inside their own walls, had to wear masks and eat and sleep alone. As they headed off to their next shifts, they often took with them their neighbors' curses, their partners' anger, and their children's fears that they would get sick and die. As one nurse put it, "It was as hard as it gets!"

Even though the SARS outbreak has been over for several years, the damage lingers. Although no one really knows the depth of trauma that still haunts patients and families from that period, many staff will privately admit to suffering from post-traumatic stress. One hospital had a psychiatrist who would meet with the staff most affected every day during the crisis and debrief with them, but staff from another hospital had no support at all—not during the outbreak or since. "We're professionals. We're supposed to be tough. We love what we do and we went into health care to help people. We learned that we have to help one another at times like this. But the emotional burden of dealing with this is huge." Some quietly express fears about possible future outbreaks of infectious diseases: "I think some staff will just refuse to come to work, and then where will we be?"

For those committed to family-centered care, it has been additionally difficult to hear some of their colleagues say how much they enjoyed not having what they called the "noise and chaos" of having family members around during SARS, that they found it more peaceful to work. As families return to the hallways of these hospitals and staff adjust to the increased traffic, hopefully too will come the reminders that patient recovery, competence, and satisfaction are all increased with the information, support, and presence of families respected for their contributions.

One team of nurses and social workers put it this way: "Certainly SARS showed that in a time of crisis, elements of care we value can be easily lost or destroyed. We are passionate about family-centered care. Even under the best of circumstances, it can be difficult to implement. We have worked long and hard to change the culture of our hospital. The fruits of our labors disappeared overnight, and the road back is proving to be tenuous. The challenge now is for leaders in health care to ensure that policies and systems are in place to allow us to respond to a public health crisis without sacrificing the relationships among patients, families, and health care providers."

The word *pandemic* is commonplace in the news of the day, and the world feels somewhat endangered. Consequently, the lessons learned and questions raised by SARS are timely and present a great opportunity for reflection and evaluation. The SARS experience provides an informed basis for planning for the future and, as such, it would be almost unethical to make plans that do not address the emotional side effects of family separation and patient isolation.

In the words of one hospital team, "We need to fully understand the cost/benefit of isolation procedures and find answers to questions such as:

- How restrictive do limits on contact between professionals and patients and families need to be?
- Might the steady presence of a family member naturally reduce the number of contacts while helping the patient and providing support for overworked staff?
- How restrictive does access to the hospital need to be?
- How widespread is the need to use protective equipment?
- How do we use families as advisors to help us answer these questions?
- What support network needs to be in place for staff and their families?"

A lesson learned from the SARS experience is that there must be proactive planning to provide appropriate support for all those who are directly affected in such public health emergencies—from public health officials and health care professionals to patients and their families. There's no question that the first priority in these situations is to protect the safety of people and control the spread of an outbreak. At the same time, however, it is also important to find ways not to abandon the standards of family-centered care and to ensure that post-traumatic stress be averted or treated.

Now is the time to plan for "the next infectious disease emergency." It is essential to bring many different points of view to the table to find the best ways to respond—including public health and infection control specialists charged with protecting public safety, patients and family members, hospital leaders, and those front-line staff who tried their best to deliver compassionate care. It is only through such an inclusive collaboration that the full ramifications of the SARS crisis will be addressed, innovative solutions will be suggested, and responsive systems will be put in place to sustain and support patients, families, and staff.

• • • • •

Government officials, infection control specialists, public health personnel, hospital leaders, and front-line staff caught in the vortex of the SARS experience were faced with phenomenal and frightening uncertainty. They were called upon to demonstrate tremendous courage, day in and day out. They are to be praised for caring, coping, and finding creative ways to adapt clinical practice in a climate of such restrictions. Their wish is that others "get ready."

This SARS story is the result of many conversations with and contributions from staff from different Toronto hospitals and infection control specialists in the United States.

If Anyone Asks,
You're Twelve-Year-Old Twins!

It was January 18, 2011, a seemingly ordinary day in Annapolis, Maryland, except for the ice storm that rolled in the night before turning a three-day weekend into a four-day weekend for our children because schools were closed. The kids, ages nine and eleven, were at home, sleeping in. My husband was just down the road at our new house, working to get it ready for us to move in. That day he was trying to fix a leak in the attic. Painters were busy downstairs.

I was at work that Tuesday morning, participating in a meeting with a board committee. My phone rang several times but, given that I was in a meeting, I ignored it. Eventually, one of the executive secretaries interrupted the meeting to tell me that my husband had been injured and I had to go to the hospital right away.

Needless to say, I was rattled especially when I learned that his injuries were so severe that he was heading to the Level 1 Trauma Center in Baltimore. A colleague drove me to the hospital and, en route, I was able to put together the pieces of what had happened and make arrangements for my children. It turns out that my husband, Mike, had plummeted twenty-four feet, falling through the drywall, shattering his feet, and generating bilateral compound pilon fractures. Fortunately, the painters were there and called 911.

Not knowing what I would be facing, I made plans for our kids to stay with a neighbor for the day. I didn't tell them anything at this point—just that I'd be home, like always, at the end of the day.

At the hospital, the orthopedic trauma team was superb and immediately stabilized my husband's legs with external fixation and traction. The doctors said we had to wait until the swelling subsided enough for major surgery to take place. He eventually had two back-to-back days in surgery—the first day was nine hours on his right leg, and the next day was seven hours on his left leg.

On the day of the accident, I got home at 6 p.m. I told the kids "Dad's had a pretty bad accident. It's probably best if we don't all visit for a couple of days to give him a chance to rest and heal." In truth, I didn't want them to see their dad in the early days because he looked pretty gruesome. I tried to assure them he'd be okay and told them that their grandparents and my sister were on their way to help out.

By the first week in February, Mike had been discharged to a rehabilitation unit and readmitted to the hospital for the two major operations. He was in the Stepdown Unit of the ICU (intensive care unit), and I felt it was okay for the kids to visit. February 6th was Super Bowl Sunday. Our family tradition was to watch the game together, often hosting a party for family and friends, so we started to plan to be together—just the four of us—on that Sunday.

My son is a huge football fan and loves the Green Bay Packers (second to the Redskins), who would be playing against the Pittsburgh Steelers. This contributed to the mounting excitement for the trip to the hospital to watch the game and see their dad. As it turned out, we would be four of the 111 million people who would watch the game that evening!

Sunday finally arrived. Complete with snacks, chips, drinks, and brownies, the three of us piled into the car. As we entered the hospital lobby and headed toward the unit, I recalled the signs outside the unit that said ABSOLUTELY NOBODY UNDER THE AGE OF 12. For a moment, I panicked and then the wheels starting turning in my head.

I spun around and said, "Kids, listen to me. This is really important. If anyone asks, you are twelve-year-old twins. Got it?" My eleven-year-old son never missed a beat and replied "Okay, Mom—so I was born on August 24, 1998, not 1999, right?" My daughter, on the other hand, looked confused and said, "When was I born?"

We quickly helped her with the math, carried on our way, and had a fabulous evening together as a family (the Packers defeated the Steelers—final score, 31 to 25). As it turned out, no one ever asked about the kids, so we never actually lied, but we had our story ready.

By the way, when my cell phone rings today, I answer it!

· · · · ·

Tori Bayless is the president and chief executive officer of Anne Arundel Medical Center in Annapolis, Maryland. She commented that the whole experience with her husband's injury, hospitalizations, surgery, and rehab—beyond worrying and then reveling in his recovery— strengthened her conviction about the importance of the patient- and family-centered journey they had begun at Anne Arundel. Welcoming families 24/7 according to the preferences of the patient was central to the change in organizational culture they were making. She said, "For me there was no looking back."

It's Not about Time:
Small Moments and Lasting
Memories

"When serious illness strikes, each one of us wants not simply
the best possible care for our body but for our whole being."
—*Kenneth B. Schwartz*

"Watch your thoughts; they become words.
Watch your words; they become actions.
Watch your actions; they become habits.
Watch your habits; they become your character.
Watch your character; it becomes your destiny."
—*Frank Outlaw*

"You may never know what results come from your
action. But if you do nothing, there will be no result."
—*Gandhi*

It's not just what happens, it's also how things happen.
It's not just what you do, but how you are. It's not
simply about techniques, treatments, and technology;
it's also about genuine, authentic, compassionate
communication and relationships.

Think about the impact of . . . a smile . . . a hug . . .
holding a hand . . . seeing past a bandage to look at
the world with a patient's eyes . . . a warm look, a kind
gesture . . . sharing tears . . . the briefest pause in the
frenetic pace of a day . . . as opposed to . . . being left
alone in a time of crisis . . . being callously dismissed
at a time of stress . . . having no one notice your pain
or your tears . . . overhearing disturbing conversations
about you and your prognosis . . ."

Everyday Gifts

When Loss Is Suppressed or Acknowledged

Simple Sentences

Making the Unbearable Bearable

She Sang Him His Life

The Magic of Music

Thanks for the Good Seats

Within a Single Day

Our Last Father's Day

Everyday Gifts

The Lady in Red

I recall getting on the elevator and joining a man and a woman. She was wearing a red outfit and a turban under which I could tell she had no hair and was on active therapy. Her face broke into a glorious smile as she said, "Good morning!" As she moved next to me, I realized she was standing behind her husband, hugging his waist, grimacing in severe pain. Yet as she began to exit the elevator, she smiled again and said, "Have a nice day!" She came to the hospital that day with courage, faith, and hope, and her very being was a testament to the strength of the human spirit.

Coaching

Scott was thirty-five and a wrestling coach, diagnosed with colorectal cancer. Two years after surgery and extraordinary health care journeys, he was invited to talk to a group of professionals to provide a patient's view of the discharge process. Later, reflecting on his talk, he said, "I've just done the most important thing in my life. It is such a privilege to help others."

9/11

The day after planes hit the World Trade Center and the Pentagon, our waiting room was full of people needing care. For them, their illnesses were their disasters, and they needed us to function. It was an awesome experience to try to put ourselves in their shoes and get past the news. I was reminded that day of a proverb that says, "He who plants a garden has faith in tomorrow." We were gardeners that day.

·····

These reflections come from a senior hospital administrator who says, "If we just pay attention, our patients give us gifts every day. They are at the center of everything we do."

When Loss Is Suppressed
or Acknowledged

Everything felt new. We'd been married for three years and had decided to move to a new city and a new country. We knew only two people when we arrived in May 1976. And then we got pregnant. It was June.

The excitement of having our first child changed to worry when the baby stopped moving. Worry changed to deep sorrow when the doctor told us, during a regular check-up at four months, that the baby was no longer alive in my uterus. He said it would be safest to allow my body to go into labor naturally when it chose to do so. It was September.

When people looked at us and said, "Oh, you're pregnant, dear—how wonderful—when are you due?" we simply smiled meekly and walked away. And we waited.

Things that needed doing were put on hold. Finally my husband had to go and close up our cottage. A couple of hours after he left, in the early evening, I went into labor. It was November.

An old family friend, a woman who had lost several babies herself, took me to the hospital. When I got there, a doctor examined me. Noticing my anxiety and fear, he glibly said, while examining me, "What are you so upset about?"

The hospital said they didn't have a bed for me and, even though I was bleeding, were going to send me home. My friend was madder than a hornet and told them that I was staying right there! I think I would have been completely neglected if she hadn't been with me. Sadly, she couldn't stay.

I was alone all night and in labor for nine hours. Then the labor pains stopped. At 6 a.m., I had to go to the bathroom. It didn't seem normal. It felt like I had passed something. I called the nurse. She looked and said, "Oh, it's just a clot." She flushed the toilet.

It was our baby.

I remember that New Year's. We went to our cottage. We stood outside and listened to the sound of the ocean. The night was dark. We were two lost souls, mired, separately, in deep grief. We didn't speak. We were young and didn't have a lot of skills or resources to deal with this experience.

I shut down emotionally for years.

• • • • •

Even though this couple went on to have three children, it took them a long time to fully understand the damage done by a single, thoughtless sentence and single thoughtless act. Ten years after the death of their first child, they decided to acknowledge his existence in their lives. They named him Matthew. As a family, with their three children, they built a small box and each of them put something into the box. With time and a lot of work on their own, they had come to a place of peace.

And then, in 2013, they received a phone call from their oldest daughter who was six months pregnant with her second child. Their daughter was crying and said, "I'm at the hospital and there's no heartbeat. Our baby has died." They flew to be with her, her husband, and their grandchild right away, arriving within twenty-four hours.

• • • • •

Our daughter had been given a choice of inducing labor, which had not been offered to me. Their baby was born the next morning. When we first saw our daughter, she was holding her tiny son and looked very peaceful. The staff couldn't have been kinder, giving us lots of time and space to be together. And when they took the baby, they held him with reverence.

Our daughter and husband and grandchild were presented with a memory box, with pictures, a little hat their baby had worn, a small bear, and his identification bracelet. Our granddaughter went through the box every day for a number of days, proudly proclaiming, "I'm already a big sister." We had a simple service at home and then another one in the summer when our son-in-law's parents and our daughter's siblings could be present. We were together as a loving and supportive family, and we buried the baby's ashes in a special "treasure chest" along with a baseball and a long letter from his mother.

What a difference between the two experiences, separated by more than thirty-five years. This time, the baby's life was acknowledged. Grief and loss were acknowledged rather than suppressed. Resources for coping were offered. When the parents were asked if they wanted to go to the crematorium, they answered, "We don't want to miss one step of this."

Simple Sentences

Egypt?

The news was not good. Andrea thought that she had beaten her breast cancer, but the doctor had just finished telling her and her husband that she now had a brain tumor.

Andrea and her husband had been planning a special trip to Egypt. She asked her doctor, "Do you think we can still go?" He answered, "It depends on where you want to die."

.....

Andrea did not go to Egypt but lived for several more months.

The Receptionist's Call

Hilary began to feel sick in midsummer. Her doctor sent her for some tests, and the early results, combined with her symptoms, suggested pancreatic cancer. She was scheduled for a fine-needle biopsy that would provide more detailed information. The procedure turned out to be a terrible experience because it took three times for the technician to "get enough cells." Hilary said she felt like a beaten-up sack of potatoes by the time it was over.

Hilary knew that the results of the biopsy would determine if the surgeon thought he could operate. She also understood that surgery would really be her only chance for, if not a cure, at least some time. She waited for the doctor to call. And then the phone rang. It was the doctor's receptionist, who simply said, "I'm calling to tell you that the surgeon will not be operating at this time."

.....

Hilary valued every day she had and described every moment she had as precious. She was in her garden two days before she died, two months after the phone call.

Overheard

When my mum was ninety-seven, she was admitted to the hospital with pneumonia. A doctor came into her room to report the results of the X-rays. He presumed that my mother was asleep and spoke directly to me: "The diagnosis isn't good. At that age, they often don't survive."

· · · · ·

When the doctor left, the older woman grinned and said to her daughter, "You tell him I'm not dead yet!"

Making the Unbearable Bearable

I had spent a considerable part of my career as a health care lawyer, first in state government and then in the private sector. I came to know a lot about health care policy and management, government regulations, and contracts. I knew little about the delivery of care, however. All that changed on November 7, 1994, when, at age forty, I was diagnosed with advanced lung cancer. In the months that followed, I was subjected to chemotherapy, radiation, surgery, and news of all kinds—most of it bad. It has been a harrowing experience for me and for my family. And yet, the ordeal has been punctuated by moments of exquisite compassion. I have been the recipient of an extraordinary array of human and humane responses to my plight. These acts of kindness—the simple human touch from my caregivers—have made the unbearable bearable.

During September and October of 1994, I made several visits to the outpatient clinic of a Boston teaching hospital for treatment of a persistent cough, low-grade fever, malaise, and weakness. The nurse practitioner diagnosed me as having atypical pneumonia and prescribed an antibiotic. Despite continued abnormal blood counts, she assured me that I had a post-viral infection and didn't need an appointment with my physician until mid-November, if then. By mid-October, I felt so bad that I decided I could not wait until November 11 to be seen. Disappointed with the inaccessibility of my physician, I decided to seek care elsewhere, with the hope that a new doctor might be more responsive.

My brother, a physician who had trained at Massachusetts General Hospital (MGH), arranged for an immediate appointment with Dr. Jose Vega, an experienced internist affiliated with the MGH. Dr. Vega spent an hour with me and ordered tests, including a chest X-ray. He called within hours to say he was concerned by the results, which showed a mass in my right lung, and he ordered a computerized tomography scan for more detail. I remember leaving my office for home, saying quickly to my secretary, Sharyn Wallace, "I think I may have a serious medical problem." Indeed, the CT scan confirmed abnormal developments in my right lung and chest nodes.

The next day, Dr. Vega, assuring me that he would continue to be available to me whenever I needed him, referred me to Dr. Thomas Lynch, a thirty-four-year-old MGH oncologist specializing in lung cancer. Dr. Lynch, who seems driven by the ferocity of the disease he sees every day, told me that I had lung cancer, lymphoma, or some rare lung infection, although it was most likely lung cancer.

My family and I were terrified. For the next several months, my blood pressure, which used to be a normal 124 over 78, went to 150 over 100, and my heart rate, which used to be a low 48, ran around 100.

Within seventy-two hours of seeing Dr. Lynch, I was scheduled for a bronchoscopy and a mediastinoscopy—exploratory surgical procedures to confirm whether I indeed had lung cancer. Until this point, I had thought that I was at low risk for cancer: I was relatively young, I did not smoke (although I had smoked about a cigarette a day in college and in law school and for several years after that), I worked out every day, and I avoided fatty foods.

The day before surgery, I was scheduled to have a series of tests. The presurgical area of the hospital was mobbed, and the nurses seemed harried. Eventually, a nurse who was to conduct a presurgical interview called my name. Already apprehensive, I was breathing hard.

The nurse was cool and brusque, as if I were just another faceless patient. But once the interview began, and I told her that

I had just learned that I probably had advanced lung cancer, she softened, took my hand, and asked how I was doing. We talked about my two-year-old son, Ben, and she mentioned that her nephew was named Ben. By the end of our conversation, she was wiping tears from her eyes and saying that while she normally was not on the surgical floor, she would come to see me before the surgery. Sure enough, the following day, while I was waiting to be wheeled into surgery, she came by, held my hand, and, with moist eyes, wished me luck.

This small gesture was powerful; my apprehension gave way to a much-needed moment of calm. Looking back, I realize that in a high-volume setting, the high-pressure atmosphere tends to stifle a caregiver's inherent compassion and humanity. But the briefest pause in the frenetic pace can bring out the best in a caregiver and do much for a terrified patient.

The nurse left, and my apprehension mounted. An hour later, I was wheeled to surgery for a biopsy of the chest nodes and the mass in my lung. I was greeted by a resident in anesthesiology, Dr. Debra Reich, who took my pulse and blood pressure and said gently, "You're pretty nervous, huh?" She medicated me with tranquilizers, but that did not stop me from asking where she lived, where she had trained, and whether she was married. I jokingly asked her how come she was the only Jewish doctor I had met during my time at MGH. When it turned out that she lived down the street from me and liked the sandwiches at the same corner shop, Virginia's, I felt comforted. She squeezed my shoulder, wished me luck, and wheeled me into surgery.

When I awoke, I was told that I had adenocarcinoma in my right lung and in several chest nodes—in other words, advanced lung cancer. I don't remember a lot about those hours, but I remember Dr. Vega's face with tears in his eyes. I also remember feeling very sad and scared.

A few days later, I received a letter from Dr. Reich:

Remember me, your friendly anesthesiologist? I came by to see you this afternoon as my professional duty but also to express my sadness in hearing about your diagnosis. Your door was closed and there seemed to be a lot of activity, so I decided not to disturb you.

As I'm sure you know, we as physicians are taught not to become emotionally involved in our patients because then we would be continually devastated. But I guess because we had such a nice interaction before your surgery and because your life was one which I could relate to so well-being Jewish, professional, renovating a house, sandwiches at Virginia's, etc.-your situation really struck a chord in me. (Hey, maybe you can't even remember any of this because of the medicine I gave you, but hopefully you do.)

I was impressed that during the fear and anxiety you were experiencing, you still maintained your composure, your sense of humor, and even thought to ask me when I was getting married.

So anyway, as you told me, keeping your wife and son in mind will make you fight strong, and I know this to be true! I know that you have a very loving and supportive family who will help you through this as well.

-Best wishes, and maybe I'll run into you sometime at Virginia's.

I had not forgotten Dr. Reich, nor will I ever forget her willingness to cross the professional barrier, hold my hand, and write those words.

It was clear that I would soon begin a new chapter in my illness and undergo the classic treatment for such advanced cancer: intensive chemotherapy and radiation, followed by surgery to remove the tumors, the nodes, and the entire lung, if necessary. Dr. Lynch told me that this option presented the real possibility of a cure.

Over the next week, I had a series of additional radiologic scans to determine if the cancer had spread beyond my chest. These scans are incredibly scary: You are placed in a tube resembling a sarcophagus, with only six inches between you and the walls, and you may spend several hours inside, deafened by the clanging machine. And the scans always raise fears about whether more bad news is around the corner.

Dr. Vega or Dr. Lynch always made it a point, though, to relay results within twenty-four hours, so my family and I didn't have to endure the anxiety of uncertainty any longer than necessary.

The scans of my body, head, liver, bones, and back were clear. I was relieved.

The doctors soon began an intensive regimen of chemotherapy and radiation, with the goal of destroying the cancer and preparing for surgery to remove my lung.

Before being admitted for my first five-day course of chemotherapy, I had a radiation-simulation session. During such sessions, therapists meticulously map their targets by marking your skin where the radiation should be directed. I was asked to lie on a table in a large, cold chamber. The radiation therapist, Julie Sullivan, offered me a blanket and, mentioning that the staff had a tape deck, asked if I had any requests. I recalled my college days and asked for James Taylor. Listening to "Sweet Baby James" and "Fire and Rain," I thought back to a time when the most serious problem I faced was being jilted by a girlfriend, and tears ran down my cheeks. As therapists came and went, Julie Sullivan held my hand and asked me if I was okay. I thanked her for her gentleness.

After having a Port-o-Cath implanted in my chest—a device that allows chemotherapy to be administered without constant needle sticks in the arm—I was admitted to MGH in mid-November. During that and other hospitalizations, either my mother or sister would stay overnight, often sleeping in cramped chairs. When I awoke at night in an anxious sweat or nauseated, I would see one of them and feel reassured.

While doctors managed my medical care, my day-to-day quality of life and comfort were in the hands of two or three nurses. These nurses showed competence and pride in their work, but they also took a personal interest in me. It gave me an enormous boost, and while I do not believe that hope and comfort alone can overcome cancer, they certainly made a huge difference to me during my time in the hospital.

During the period between my two chemotherapies, when I also received high-dose radiation twice a day, I came to know a most exceptional caregiver, the outpatient oncology nurse Mimi Bartholomay. An eight-year veteran who had experienced cancer in her own family, she was smart, upbeat, and compassionate. I had to receive fluids intravenously every day at the clinic, and while I was there, we talked regularly about life, cancer, marriage, and children. She, too, was willing to cross that professional Rubicon—to reach out and talk about my fear of dying or, even worse, my fear of not living out my life, of not biking through the hills of Concord and Weston on summer weekends with my brother, of not seeing my child grow up, of not holding my wife in my arms. And she took the risk of talking about her own father's recent bout with cancer. I cannot emphasize enough how meaningful it was to me when caregivers revealed something about themselves that made a personal connection to my plight. It made me feel much less lonely. The rule books, I'm sure, frown on such intimate engagement between caregiver and patient. But maybe it's time to rewrite them.

After my second round of chemotherapy, I was ready for the final stage of what we hoped would be a cure: surgery. Before this could happen, Dr. Lynch repeated my radiologic scans to be sure that the cancer had not spread. He assured me that the chance of any such metastasis was remote—less than 5 percent—although it would be a disaster if it occurred.

The scans were endless, scary, and lonely. While members of my family stayed with me in the waiting rooms, they could not accompany me to the scanning rooms; the experience again was harrowing. But I felt my greatest fear while awaiting the results. After a week of tests, I had one last scan of my bones. I was concerned when the technologist asked to do a special scan of my back that had not been done before.

The next day, I called Dr. Lynch's office and asked his assistant, Mary Ellen Rousell, when I could come in to find out the results. She said, "How about this afternoon?" and then added, "You might want to bring someone." My heart skipped. When my wife and I entered Dr. Lynch's office and saw his face, our hearts sank. He was ashen. He said that while all the other scans were clear, there appeared to be a metastatic tumor in my spine. He explained that this meant that lung surgery at this point would be futile, since other metastases were likely to surface.

Dr. Lynch said that he could not be 100 percent certain that this was a tumor and that, because so much was at stake, we should do a biopsy. My wife and I wept openly—in part, because, looking at Dr. Lynch's face, we felt that he had lost hope.

I could not help but ask what treatment options were available, and he mentioned a drug called Taxol. Still being the lawyer, I quizzed him:

> ME: What is the percentage of people who benefit from Taxol?
>
> DR. LYNCH: Forty percent.
>
> ME: How much do they benefit?
>
> DR. LYNCH: They can get several years of life, although it is not a cure. And the median survival for patients on Taxol with your advanced stage of disease is nine months.

Nine months! My wife and I cringed. I ended the session by asking Dr. Lynch, "How do you do this work?" And he answered, in genuine pain, "By praying that I don't have days like today."

I began to have trouble sleeping, and when I awoke, I was filled with dread and despair. I thought frequently of the observation of Richard Block, the founder of H&R Block, who had survived lung cancer after being told initially that he had only months to live: "I lived for five days without hope and . . . my life during those five days . . . was far worse than at any time during the 'horrible' ordeal of tests and treatments."

And when I contemplated not living to see my son grow up or not cherishing my wife for a lifetime, I thought of King Lear, who, at a low point, wailed:

I am bound

Upon a wheel of fire, that mine own tears

Do scald like molten lead.

A few days later, I had the biopsy. Dr. Lynch met with my family to report that, indeed, after considerable searching, the pathologist had found small deposits of adenocarcinoma in my vertebra. It was now confirmed that I had metastatic lung cancer. Although my brother and my father, who is also a physician, raised the possibility of radical surgery on my back and lung to remove all the tumors, Dr. Lynch and the surgeons rejected this option because further metastases were likely to appear, and the surgery would be debilitating and reduce my quality of life at a time when my life could well be substantially shortened.

The clear treatment was more chemotherapy. Dr. Lynch again recommended the use of Taxol, with the hope of slowing the cancer's spread.

My wife and I were largely silent during the medical discussion. I asked my father and brother to leave so that my wife and I could talk not facts and figures but matters of the heart. When they had left, I said to Dr. Lynch, "You told me two things all along: One, that you were aiming for a total cure, and if that were not feasible, you would tell me at that time. And two, you would never, ever give up on me, never stop trying to fight, to extend my life as long as possible. Am I no longer on the cure route?"

He looked somberly at us and explained that there were no known treatments to cure this stage of cancer.

"And will you stick by me and fight to the end?" I asked.

He nodded vigorously and then outlined a number of state-of-the-art, experimental protocols from which I might benefit after Taxol.

And leaving statistics behind, he talked of several patients who had defied the odds and lived for years beyond expectations. He advised that my goal should be to be here the same time next year, and then the year after, and the year after—one day at a time. He mentioned several breast cancer patients who had told him that they had relished their final years with their children in a way that they had never known before. It felt good to leave the medical talk and speak heart to heart, and it felt to me that he had regained a sense of hope—not for some magical cure, but for the possibility of extending my life.

It was crucial to my wife and to me that he not give up hope. I understood his surprise and disappointment at the metastases; in fact, as one friend suggested, his distress at that event was a sign of his caring about me and his involvement with my case. But we desperately needed him to give us a realistic basis for hope—and he had.

The next day, I began a new chapter in my fight. And once again, Mimi Bartholomay was by my side, monitoring my reaction and assuring me that most people tolerated Taxol very well. I had no allergic reaction, and I felt good that the battle was underway. I had hoped that maybe this could buy me time.

Time was now my best friend, since it could allow medical research to advance and doctors to find new strategies and maybe even a cure for advanced lung cancer.

During this period, with help from my father, who has had a long and distinguished career in academic medicine, I began to explore potential cutting-edge protocols that could supplement or follow Taxol.

My father arranged a meeting for my wife and me with Dr. Kurt J. Isselbacher, a distinguished researcher and director of the MGH Cancer Center. He is a small man with a large presence and piercing blue eyes, and he was surrounded by medical books, papers, and many pictures of his family. He was upbeat, telling us of protocols underway that showed promise in fighting metastatic tumors. Like several others, he told me a personal story that cut to the bone: A close family member, he said, had been diagnosed with advanced cancer, which the attending oncologist had said was "very, very bad." The family member had said to him, "Kurt, you have helped so many people in your life; can you now help me?" He personally treated the family member in that person's home with chemotherapy, and, twenty-one years later, that person is thriving.

Dr. Isselbacher offered to serve as an advocate for me, to work with my father and Dr. Lynch to find the most promising protocols. I told him at the meeting that while I had no illusions, I was deeply moved by his refusal to give up and by his abiding hope. I was especially affected because such hopefulness was not coming from a faith healer, but from a distinguished researcher. He had strengthened our resolve to fight.

As I grappled to maintain my hope in the face of the advancing disease, I was referred to Dr. Ned Cassem, a senior MGH psychiatrist who not only had had vast experience with the seriously ill, but was himself a Jesuit priest. I had met with him once during my second hospitalization, and my memory through the haze was that he was the first person with whom I had discussed death. I remembered that when I asked him if, when, and how I should say good-bye to people, he said, "You know, you don't have to wait to say good-bye; you can express your love and appreciation for people right now, every day."

After the devastating news of the metastases, I felt the urge to seek out Dr. Cassem again, in part to ask if there was anything more I should be doing to help my son, Ben, cope with my illness or the eventuality of my death. I mentioned that several people had suggested I make a videotape for Ben, but I thought I couldn't do that. Dr. Cassem replied that every time we played or laughed together, we were creating building blocks, precious memories that will be a part of him forever.

I also asked him if he thought I should be doing more to prepare for the possibility of an early death. He looked perplexed and asked, "Have you prepared your will?" I said yes. "Are your affairs otherwise in order?" I again said yes. "So it sounds like you are prepared. Remember, death is a minor matter. Living . . . that's the challenge."

I then told him of the paradox that moments of great pleasure—playing with my son, snuggling with my wife, talking intensely with friends—also caused me great pain and tears. Was I depressed? Was this something to worry about? He looked at me thoughtfully and said, "When you cry about your son, it's because he has touched you deeply. It's an affirmation of your love for him. When you weep about the joy you experienced with your wife or close friends, that's an acknowledgment of your love for them. That's not a bad thing. Maybe a day without tears has been a dull day." I nodded and then could not help but ask, "Do you believe in the power of prayer?" Dr. Cassem nodded. "Absolutely," he said, "and your name is on my prayer list." I felt warmed in his presence, by his wisdom, his common sense, and his spirituality.

In recent months, I have had several setbacks: a bone scan that showed four to five additional tumors and a CT scan that showed significant progression of the cancer in both lungs. The only good news was that it had not spread to my head or liver. I am pained, but not surprised, at the relentlessness of the disease, and I am straining to retain hope that one of the experimental treatments may succeed where chemotherapy has failed.

For the first time, I recently mentioned to Dr. Lynch the idea of a hospice service and wondered how I might reduce future pain as the cancer progresses. Dr. Lynch answered that we were still a long way from that discussion, that we still had many avenues to explore, and that he remained as committed as ever to doing whatever he could to extend my life in a quality way.

Around the time of the CT scan, when I was feeling particularly dejected, I had an appointment with Mimi Bartholomay for an injection. She was running late, and as she approached me in the clinic, she looked harried. But as she got closer, she could see how unhappy I was, and she put her arm around me and directed me to a private room. I began to cry, and she intuitively responded, "You know, scan days are the worst. But whatever the results, we are not going to give up on you. We're going to fight with you and for you all the way." I hugged her and thanked her for hanging in there with me.

If I have learned anything, it is that we never know when, how, or whom a serious illness will strike. If and when it does, each one of us wants not simply the best possible care for our body, but for our whole being.

I am still bound upon Lear's wheel of fire, but the love and devotion of my family and friends, and the deep caring and engagement of my caregivers, have been a tonic for my soul and have helped to take some of the sting from my scalding scars.

In my new role as a patient, I have learned that medicine is not merely about performing tests or surgeries, or administering drugs. These functions, important as they are, are just the beginning. For as skilled and knowledgeable as my caregivers are, what matters the most is that they have empathized with me in a way that gives me hope and makes me feel like a human being, not just an illness.

Again and again, I have been touched by the smallest kind gestures—a squeeze of my hand, a gentle touch, a reassuring word. In some ways, these quiet acts of humanity have felt more healing than the high-dose radiation and chemotherapy that hold the hope of a cure.

As an eminent Harvard Medical School professor, himself a cancer patient, once taught, "The secret of the care of the patient is caring for the patient."

.....

Kenneth B. Schwartz died of lung cancer in September 1995. Shortly before his death, The Kenneth B. Schwartz Center at Massachusetts General Hospital was founded, which is dedicated to strengthening the relationship between patients and caregivers.

This story, by Kenneth B. Schwartz, originally appeared in The Boston Globe Magazine *on July 16, 1995, under the title "A Patient's Story." With minor changes to reflect the passage of time, it is reprinted here with the permission of The Kenneth B. Schwartz Center (now called The Schwartz Center for Compassionate Healthcare).*

She Sang Him His Life

Palliative care seems to be a place where anything goes. On our unit, the hours are completely open; people come and go as they need; pets visit. Staff pay attention to so many little details of comfort. There's a tenderness and kindness on the unit that's extraordinary. By comparison, when I visit someone on another floor, it's impersonal, and I feel assaulted by noise, unpleasant smells, and a sense of crowdedness.

One night, I arrived for my regular volunteer shift on the palliative care unit and found the staff in a very emotional state. This was not entirely unusual, but I sensed that something special had happened that day. I was right.

A young man, in his early forties, had been on the unit for several days. His wife had been with him almost constantly. This husband and wife were both from the same tiny village in Newfoundland. They had grown up together, become a couple, gotten married, and lived there all their lives. And now this man, her husband, was dying.

She knew that the end was near and asked the nurses if she could get into bed with her husband and snuggle. And the answer was, "Of course you can, dear."

And then the singing started. It went on for well over an hour. This woman, as she cuddled her dying husband, slowly and gently, sang him his life and their lives together.

When the singing stopped, her husband was still alive. She then she sang him permission to leave.

●●●●●

When asked why this woman chose to become a volunteer in palliative care, she explained that it was because of her experience with her father. When he was dying, in a different hospital and far away, she says that the care he received in palliative care was so dear that she told herself, "This is what I'm going to do someday."

The Magic of Music

Music for me is like magic. When I go to the extendicare center where I work part-time, what I see when I walk in are so many old people, sitting in wheelchairs. They are not doing anything, not saying anything, not noticing anyone or anything around them. But then I start to play and sing songs from the 1920s and 1930s. Toes begin tapping, then I hear a gentle humming followed by tentative words, and soon, the whole room has come alive. People sing and talk to one another, sharing stories about memories evoked by the music.

Staff participate as well. The music appears to be therapy for them, too. They seem more excited about the work they're doing and the people they're working with. They see that behind the usual blank stares, there are people with rich past lives.

There's one woman I work with on a one-to-one basis because she has a bad back and it's hard for her to sit. When I go in to see her, she's usually sprawled across her bed, dozing. I gently nudge her awake and she gets very excited. I play songs such as "Frankie and Johnny" and "Five Foot Two" for her because she knows all the words and sings right along. She sits right up and waves her arms in rhythm with the music. When I have to leave, she always says, "Please don't go. Please don't go." I feel guilty because there's generally a lethargic feeling in the air and not much incentive to be active or intellectually stimulated.

I also work on a psychiatric unit with people from ages eighteen to eighty. My goal is to provide a joyful and magical experience for everyone through music making and improvisation. Music is a great vehicle for socializing and having a good time, breaking down age barriers, and providing some positive distraction from worries. Two particular experiences stand out in my mind.

One night, I remember singing James Taylor's "Fire and Rain," which has the words "I always knew I'd see you again" in reference to someone who has died. One of the women who was in the hospital for depression started to cry. It turned out that her husband had recently died. She thanked me, saying that crying felt like a great release. She then asked if she could have a copy of the words. When I returned, I brought her a copy of the lyrics. She was so surprised and delighted that I had remembered.

Another time, a cluster of young patients in their twenties, very much part of the rave scene, asked me to bring in some progressive house and trance music. When I did, the young kids started dancing while the other patients watched in awe. Eventually, everyone, even the patients in their seventies, started dancing. The young people felt very positive about having contributed something enjoyable to others on the unit, and they remarked they'd had a good time. They didn't know it was possible to do so without drugs and alcohol.

It's exciting to see music helping people progress and improve. It is interesting to me that attendance on the nights when Music with Ann is offered is about 80 percent, whereas attendance for activities such as crafts, games, and outings is only 30 percent.

Tragically, music is often seen as a frill, and music therapy is usually at the bottom of the budget pile. I'll keep writing proposals, however, because I see the magic that happens with music.

•••••

Ann is a certified music therapist. Her dream job would be to work in psychiatry full-time.

Thanks for the Good Seats

We had a gentleman on our unit who had brain cancer. One night, when he seemed particularly restless, I suggested that we go to the cafeteria for tea. Ever the gentleman, he seemed worried and said, "But I don't have any money." I told him not to worry about that.

Try to picture the scene. He has a huge bandage on his head and is wearing hospital pajamas. I'm in street clothes. Once I got him comfortable in his wheelchair, the two of us set off.

It was nighttime, and there was an enormous blizzard blowing outside. The cafeteria has huge glass windows to the outside. Because it was dark outside and the cafeteria lights were on, these windows reflected the room. The reflection was not complete like a mirror, however, because you could still see the storm and the twinkling lights of the snowy parking lot.

I wasn't really paying attention to any of this as I settled my gentleman at a table. We chatted briefly about what kind of a doughnut he would like as a special treat, and I said I'd be right back. When I returned with his tea and doughnut, he looked up at me and said, "Thanks for getting us such good seats for the show." I suddenly got it—I got under his bandage and saw the world with his eyes—and, stifling my laughter, I simply said, "You're welcome."

Within a Single Day

Within a single day, I saw some of the best and the worst of current practice. My mother-in-law and I were accompanying my father-in-law to consultations with two different pulmonary oncologists. For the first visit, the three of us were taken into a room with four stretchers and only curtains for privacy. My eighty-year-old father-in-law was asked to sit on the edge of a stretcher with his legs dangling over the side. There was a chair for my mother-in-law; I stood.

When the doctor finally arrived, he did not acknowledge my mother-in-law or me. He spoke directly to my father-in-law, saying, "I talk quietly, so you will have to turn up your hearing aid." With barely a pause, he continued saying, "I've looked at the test results. You have a cancer that won't respond to treatment. There's nothing we can do for you."

He basically left us with no hope. He conveyed no feelings or concern for our experience. He failed to provide any information about what would happen. He offered no help for how we would manage in the coming days and weeks. He didn't ask us if we had any questions. It was as though my father-in-law was merely an irritating, negative test result in his busy day. The doctor walked out, leaving the three of us there alone and stunned. Although he said nothing, my father-in-law's stooped shoulders and hanging head communicated complete despair.

The afternoon encounter was another story altogether. The second doctor invited the three of us into a room with comfortable chairs, asked everyone to sit, and spoke to each of us by name, making sure he understood how we were all connected to my father-in-law. In essence, he had the same message as the morning doctor, but he delivered it quite differently. He was clear about there being no further curative interventions, but was also clear about saying, "I want to work together with you. How can I be most helpful?" He answered our questions and engaged us all in discussion. We did not feel alone and, even better, we felt we were part of a team.

I was struck by the difference between these two experiences in the same day. Although the diagnosis was still awful, there was a sense of caring and compassion offered by the afternoon doctor that made us feel supported and encouraged us to believe that we could cope. We often hear that there's no time for compassion in health care, but both of these encounters took exactly the same amount of time!

The day reinforced my belief that health care is about people, about communication and relationships, and about helping patients and families deal with difficult situations. It's not just about whether a professional can fix or not fix something.

Our Last Father's Day

It seemed in just a few short weeks, my father went from being a strong independent man who always knew best to a person reduced to a diagnosis, a set of complicated and ever-changing presentations. He became a man who was dependent on a system of care surrounding him that didn't seem to truly grasp how far removed he had become from the man I had so admired growing up.

I attempted to pay attention and absorb what was being said as his treatment team "rounded on him." It was so odd that, after all the time I had spent working as a nurse in a hospital, I didn't have a clue how the working of a hospital really appeared to patients or families. I couldn't figure out who was in charge of which part of his body. I tried my best to keep up as his health continued to deteriorate, and the amount of health care intervention continued to grow.

After knowing my father my entire life, experts began to redefine him in terms I would have never considered using to describe him: "the ARF" (shortened medical jargon for acute renal failure); "the pancreatitis in twelve." Instead of being seen as my strong, reliable father, he was now being described as "the confused, demented, elderly patient." Sometimes, perhaps as an attempt to be reassuring, we were told, "This is common for his age." For us, however, this was anything but common. For my father and my family, this was wildly uncommon and a completely unique experience.

Among my fondest childhood memories were the times spent listening to my dad's stories on our family camping trips. Our family loved to hike and camp and, during the long evenings together, I could always get him to tell stories about the places he had been while serving in the military. Though we never traveled far away, the stories my dad told transported me to a world that filled my imagination. He would recall the most intricate details, not so much of the places themselves as his impressions of them: the feel of the grass, the smell of the air, the taste of the food, and the color of the clothes people wore. I could almost feel the wind as it blew warm or cool, depending on his tale.

Perhaps his penchant for storytelling and my delight in the imaginary explains our shared fondness for old-time radio dramas. When I was a young girl, my mother went to law school at night. My dad and I would drive thirty minutes to the school and sit in the car waiting for my mother to get out of class. To pass the time, we would listen to Radio Mystery Theater with E. G. Marshall, an attempt at radio show revival during the 1970s. During the show, we would try to guess who committed the dastardly act. I would "rest my eyes" during the last fifteen minutes of the show, but my dad let me pretend I had been awake the whole time. When the show finished and we waited for my mother, we would talk about the show and explain our rationale for choosing the suspect. Almost always our conversations would wander.

I remember my dad's last Father's Day. He was in hospital, and I gave him a CD collection of old-time mystery radio shows. I think the CDs were probably more for me than for him, but, as always, he played along. I'd place a CD in a portable stereo I had brought from home. He seemed to like the idea of hearing the stories even though he couldn't really listen. He didn't feel well enough to do much other than drift in and out of sleep.

At some point on that Father's Day evening, his nurse peeked in the room and motioned to me that she would come back a little later. She quietly shut the door and, at that moment, every patient monitor, every hall conversation, every ringing telephone, and every supply cart rolling by faded into the distance. It was as if we were sitting in that dark parking lot in our family car, me and my dad and Radio Mystery Theater, just as I remembered.

When the show was over, my dad opened his eyes and said, "I knew who did it the whole time." Our roles had reversed. He had slept through the ending this time like I had so many times and so many years ago. He smirked and I giggled because we both knew he had no clue "whodunit" as he'd been fast asleep. I welcomed the familiar grin on his face as we shared our inside joke amid the disorder and chaos that now seemed to fill every aspect of our lives.

Like old times our conversations wandered. I was in graduate school at the time, so he asked me how school was going. It was my turn to reveal details of place. I told him about the fog-shrouded Millbury Student Union (UCSF Parnassus campus) and about the great library. He remembered the library and fondly called it "the crossroads of the world." My father softly told me his disappointment that no one used libraries anymore and how youth would never understand the silence of the great rooms of knowledge and the smell of old books.

The nurse came and went very quietly as we continued to talk. I don't remember why she was there, but I do recall feeling comforted when she looked at me and smiled. She was careful not to disturb the intimate conversation unfolding between her dying patient and his daughter in the dim light. She always closed the door as she left the room. Finally my, dad drifted off to sleep and, in my exhaustion, so did I.

In the days that followed, my father succumbed to his illness. Since that time, I frequently reflect on a speech that Don Berwick delivered at the 2009 International Forum on Quality and Safety in Health Care in Berlin. In that talk, he told the audience that we would all be better off, "if professionals would behave with patients and families not as their hosts in our care system, but as guests in their lives."

I'm struck by how much we track and report in our health systems. Why do we count how many patients are in our hospitals, but not how many lives we are actually touching? So many people make up our experience of living: people whom we can delight and comfort by just slowing down from our hurried pace and taking a moment to listen to them with the goal of understanding what they are telling us; people whom we can disappoint or frustrate when we assume to know what is right as we define them in our professional terms, rather than on their experiences as unique and vibrant individuals with stories and experiences that far exceed anything we will have the privilege of knowing. As health care professionals, we are able to improve patient experiences, not only through science and high-tech interventions, but also by small gestures of respect and compassion such as slowing down, staying quiet, smiling, and providing people with time to be together, perhaps for the last time. We are not hosts; we are guests in their lives.

I frequently think about the nurse who shut the door to allow my dad and me to be together. A gift from her to us—no more monitors, no more call lights, no more ringing telephones, just me and my dad and Radio Mystery Theater. She took the time. She gave us respite from the unsettling experience of being in a hospital. She gave us a moment of peace and quiet on our last Father's Day. On that night, that nurse not only cared for my father, she cared for me as well.

·····

A version of this story first appeared in Anna Roth's blog "Doing Common Things Uncommonly Well." Anna Roth is currently the chief executive officer of Contra Costa Regional Medical Center and Health Centers in the San Francisco Bay Area.

Hope for the Future:
Passion for the Possible

"Determine the thing that is to be done
and then we will find the way."
—*Abraham Lincoln*

"We are such stuff as dreams are made of."
—*William Shakespeare*

"We are not in a position in which we have
nothing to work with. We already have capacities,
talent, direction, missions, callings."
—*Abraham Maslow*

"Risk more than others think is safe.
Care more than others think is wise.
Dream more than others think is practical.
Expect more than others think is possible."
—*Cadet Maxim, US Military Academy, West Point*

"We are all waiting for an invitation to do good."
—*Gerri Frager, MD*

Hope for the future of patient- and family-centered health care is embedded in two sentinel facts: first, that any number of examples already exist of the kind of care we all hope to have . . . care that is compassionate, collaborative, and based on dignity, respect, and full, transparent communication, and second, that there are people working hard to make change and to maintain gains that have been made.

Just as the legendary phoenix rises from the ashes, often from a situation of great challenge comes something good.

Learning from Tragedy

The Capacity to Do Good

Finding Meaning in Chaos

It Doesn't Take Much

The White Coat

When the World Turns Upside Down:
A Doctor Experiences Being a Patient

The Other Side of the Bed

Behind a Locked Door

Creating a Culture

Learning from Tragedy

I joined Dana-Farber Cancer Institute (DFCI) in 1995, six months after a tragic and much publicized medication error led to the untimely death of a cancer patient who was also a well-known health columnist for the *Boston Globe*. Staff were anxious, apprehensive, insecure, and grieving. They knew we had to deliver care and were committed to that, yet they also knew everyone was looking at us and "wondering."

At the time, I believed we had a responsibility to learn everything we could about the causes of the medication error, to take steps to make sure such a mistake never happened again, then to turn the tragedy into a vision and practice of being the very best place to receive cancer care. As part of this process, we realized we needed to speak openly and honestly about what had happened and what we were going to do about it. In the first two years after the tragedy, we spoke to thousands of leaders across the country via a series of Joint Commission on Accreditation of Healthcare Organizations (JCAHO) presentations as well as many others. The support of the organization and the interest in our journey was rewarding and invigorating.

We had many areas of key learning and change in response to the tragedy. Some of the biggest changes were made around involving patients and families. I had come to DFCI from a children's hospital, where we were used to working with patients and families all the time. Yet, when I moved into adult care, I couldn't find the patients or families anywhere except in patient rooms.

I used to tell staff at DFCI that, in pediatrics, we had already learned that "there's no stronger force in the world than a parent in your face!" We also had learned how much patients and families have to offer.

I wanted to put patients and families at the center of our world. I engaged the board and key patient care leaders. We started by just listening to patients and their families and inviting them into a few processes. Many staff thought this was crazy, but within weeks they were saying, "They're teaching us things we didn't know." Within the first year, we had more than 100 patients and family members on committees.

Now we involve patients, family members, and survivors on virtually every clinical operations committee in the hospital, including search committees for senior staff, employee orientation programs, construction programs, and the quality improvement and risk management committee of the board. The involvement of patients and families has become an expectation, not an exception. I am convinced this has led to better, safer, and more respectful and compassionate clinical care and success.

There is now a profound awareness of the unique insights and advice that those who have been the recipients of care can bring to the table. Their observations and suggestions have led to a wide variety of changes that include structural improvements in renovation projects, a new fast-track system for immuncompromised patients arriving in pediatric emergency, a patient rounding program by patients and family members, supportive therapies such as massage and acupuncture, and a program in which patients teach physicians-in-training how to break bad news and how to stay connected to and ensure support for patients and families when clinical therapies have run their course. We have even cracked the hard nut of reducing waiting times in clinics and have sought their assistance in billing notices.

I believe that involving patients and families raises the quality of care and reinforces the notion of a partnership in care as suggested by the expression, "Nothing about me, without me." We need to be alerted to problems in real time, rather than having to wait for patient satisfaction surveys to be tabulated and summarized. We also need to design procedures and facilities to meet the needs of patients and families. Only they can tell us what those needs are.

For example, one day I got a call from one of our patients about the overcrowded conditions in our infusion area. I went down and met with the nurse manager, patients, and family members. Everyone agreed that the lack of patient privacy and nursing work space was unacceptable. Existing plans to renovate the unit were halted, and patients and staff gathered to reassess them. The end result is an area that is now much more respectful of and comfortable for all. I have no idea how many people that patient helped with his single phone call.

We want to make sure we are improving the right things. And we can do this only by having patients and families with us every step of the way. They remind us that we may be excellent, but we're not perfect yet!

We are blessed to have the commitment of so many people who are both wise and willing to donate their time. One of our hundreds of volunteers, Regina Mead, a former patient and employee of IBM, and now co-chair emeritus of Dana-Farber's Adult Patient and Family Advisory Committee, has said, "When I underwent treatment here, it was obvious it is about the most patient-centered organization I have ever been associated with. From the top administrators to the parking lot attendants—they are all focused on one question: What can I do to make things better for the patient? That's the kind of place I wanted to continue to be associated with."

Have patients and families given us a hard time? Yes. Have they told us things we sometimes didn't want to hear? Yes. But do they feel respected by the organization and feel heard? Yes. And have they created the impetus and provided the perspective to make this a better place? Yes . . . without a doubt!

•••••

At the time of this story, Jim Conway was executive senior vice president and chief operations officer at Dana-Farber Cancer Institute.

The Capacity to Do Good

Dr. Gerri Frager, medical director of Pediatric Palliative Care at the IWK Health Centre, crossed the courtyard. There was energy in her step. She had said she'd be wearing red shoes. Looking up from her shoes to her face, I noted her smile and felt her warmth. We found a quiet place to talk.

Q: *How did you become interested in palliative care?*

A: It was really several patients I cared for, first as a nurse and later during my internal medicine internship, who helped me understand how important this aspect of care can be. Within the first month of my internship, I knew internal medicine was not for me, and I ultimately switched to pediatrics. While doing a fellowship at Sloan Kettering in New York, I became involved in the Death in America Project, an initiative funded by George Soros to "develop innovative programs in clinical care, research, education, and advocacy to improve the care of the dying." It was an opportunity of a lifetime. Not only did I get to do my own work, I ultimately became part of a network of eighty-seven others who were doing inspiring work.

Q: *What does the term **palliative care** mean to you?*

A: Comfort, pain management, symptom management, and emotional and spiritual support.

Q: *You didn't mention death or dying or end of life.*

A: I don't think palliative care should just be available to those who are dying. There are times when a patient and family may need the elements of palliative care—comfort, pain management, symptom management—throughout an illness that will end in recovery. One shouldn't have to wait until the end of life to access this kind of care.

Q: *You are the head of a palliative care "service" rather than a "unit." What is the difference?*

A: I specifically didn't want to have a palliative care unit at this hospital for a number of reasons. The most important reason is that I think the approaches of palliative care should be available everywhere in the hospital and at all times. In this hospital, staff are already very sensitive. They provide competent, compassionate care and collaborate well with families. I don't want to be another layer. I want to work alongside others and be a resource to them.

My job is to help them in their jobs, to provide guidance and support when they come up against a new situation in which they are not quite sure what to do next. As well, for the children and families who come to our health center, and particularly for those who have chronic illnesses and come repeatedly throughout their lives, they already know the staff on their regular units. It would be counterproductive to displace children and families from those support networks and move them to a new, unfamiliar environment, especially one with a potentially "loaded" title.

If someone is in the last days or hours of his or her life, and we need more space for extended family and more privacy, we can take over a couple of rooms and create a sense of quiet on the unit where the patient and family already know the staff and their way around.

Q: *How do you support staff?*

A: They tell me and our team what they need. I can make clinical suggestions for how the management of pain and other symptoms can be improved. If they want me to do so, I will meet with patients and families, but this is never to take away their role but rather to support their work. Because this is a regional referral hospital, we also consult with staff throughout the region and in remote communities. Sometimes there are "telehealth" conferences with a child's whole care team in that community.

  I also listen. People often forget that when a child and family are suffering, the staff suffer, too, or when a child dies, the staff grieve, although in obviously very different ways and dimensions than the family. We send bereavement baskets to the unit when a child dies. The baskets contain food, quotes, pictures, candles, little gestures of comfort, and always a card affirming the work they did and acknowledging that it is tough to be the people helping at such a special time in the life of a family.

  These baskets are even sent to the outlying communities when we know that a child has died. The first time we did this, we heard, "No one has ever done something like this or thanked us before!"

  This next thing may sound simple and small, but I've been surprised by the feedback. I love taking pictures, and I also love quotes and books. I have a bulletin board outside my office, and I pick a theme every couple of months. I put together photos and quotes and make copies available for people to take away. Often people leave notes of thanks or stories about what the picture means to them. Sometimes I get new pictures and quotes back. It's about comfort and connection and communicating on a different level.

Q: *If you could provide advice to young doctors, what would you say?*

A: I would tell them that we have the capacity to do good, even when things are not going well, and not to be afraid of being a part of those situations.

Q: *Where do your compassion and kindness come from?*

A: I believe we all have this inherently in us. Someone once said we are all waiting for an invitation to do good. Sometimes it takes a personal experience to wake up this goodness. Sometimes it takes a special invitation, a specific request.

Q: *Can compassion and kindness be learned?*

A: Yes. Some people just need help and encouragement to see what they can do. There are some who test my belief, though. At times, you might have to be strategic and creative in how or when you put out the invitation to do good.

And there are some "sharks" out there who seem to be set only on destruction. It's good to be aware of sharks, but I don't want to live my life in fear of them, always looking over my shoulder. I don't want to lose my vulnerability, my soft "underbelly."

Q: *From what you know about hospitals, what would you want if you were a patient?*

A: I'd want my basic needs of warmth, shelter, and nourishment covered. I'd want to be comfortable enough to see out a window that opens so that I could breathe the air and look out at nature. I'd want some privacy and the capacity to fill my space with the people and a few small things that are meaningful to me.

Q: *You provide so much support for others. Who supports you?*

A: I make sure I get time to be outdoors, hiking, breathing fresh air, listening to birds, looking at flowers, taking pictures, and sometimes sharing that with someone close to me. Nature nourishes and restores me. I can remember a time, though, when I was involved in the care of two teenagers, back to back, whose dying was protracted, and their diseases completely challenged their independence in terrible ways.

When the second young person died, I was physically exhausted and ravaged by the emotional impact of caring for them. The injustice of their deaths felt so profound. I knew I had to get away.

I spent part of my time away, out in nature. Then I attended a week-long retreat called "Healing the Wounded Healer." It was comforting to be in the presence of others who were also feeling so human and so vulnerable. And now I'm back.

Finding Meaning in Chaos

Linda Clarke has a very long title. In addition to being a writer and storyteller, she is the facilitator of the Program in Narrative Medicine in the Medical Humanities Program of the Faculty of Medicine at Dalhousie University in Halifax, Nova Scotia. Long as the title is, though, it only hints at what she does or why she does it.

In short, Linda is trying to touch the next generation of doctors and open their minds and hearts to the power of hearing and telling stories. She passionately believes that we never feel more validated than when we are invited to share something about ourselves. Stories provide meaning, make connections, and create a sense of community—of belonging.

Linda's journey to this work is an interesting story in itself. Many factors forged Linda's passion for storytelling. It's not as simple as just understanding that she has a background in theater and training in storytelling. It's more personal than that.

Linda's work in health care began in the world of academic bioethics. While she appreciated that the field was principle driven and designed to be thoughtful and impartial, she longed to get closer to the real people and the real experiences from which ethical issues and questions were arising. This began to happen when Linda moved from a university setting to working directly in a hospital-based clinical ethics service. Working with members of the hospital community, walking the halls, catching conversations over coffee, observing and listening to the caregivers, and, in time, from her own experiences as a patient and the child of a sick father, she witnessed the power of stories firsthand.

"People are the markers of our health care institutions, and stories are the markers of people. We can't respond completely to one another from a distance. Stories are one of the ways we can enter into relationships with one another, and it is from within those relationships that we can provide good care. It is a fundamental act of caring to invite and to receive the story of another person."

Linda continues, "My father had a stroke and lost his speech. I would travel every weekend to be with him and help him navigate the health care system. It was stressful and exhausting. One Monday, when I got back to work, I heard some staff talking about dealing with a difficult family over the weekend. I wondered if they knew anything about the context of that family. I gently interjected to tell them my story. I started with, 'Let me tell you what it may be like to be in their shoes. . . .' "

Linda also frames her own experience as a patient in terms of story. When seeking a diagnosis, Linda struggled to have her story of troubling symptoms fully heard by doctors.

As so often happens in the culture of medicine, instead of being able to hear my story in my own terms, doctors would frame what I said within their own worldview. "Headaches? Well, you must be under stress. Fatigue? You're obviously working too hard."

My medical story was continuously returned to me, in ways that made sense to the doctors but did not make sense to me. Instead of working with my story, many sent me away, believing their own. I was being required to fit their stories, not the other way around. This is a classic move in the health care culture, but it can feel profoundly dismissive to the person who is ill and seeking care.

Sadly, in spite of months of specific head-related complaints, persistently and eloquently described, a cyst kept growing in the middle of Linda's brain, undiagnosed. It took a crisis before her story was fully heard and believed. "What's really frightening is that I was someone who worked in the hospital. I knew people. I knew the ropes. If I couldn't get my story heard, what happens to those who are more vulnerable—the elderly, the homeless, people from other cultures, people who do not speak English? How do we hear their stories?"

In her current role, Linda invites medical students to share stories with one another from their own lives. "They don't have to be clever. The medical humanities program, which my work is part of, is not only about creativity. It's about building a context for understanding both yourself and your patients and your community."

Through work with story, students experience firsthand that asking for people's stories makes them feel valued in their entirety. They hear, in their own stories and in the stories of others, not only what happened, but also what was important. Stories help them get to know one another on a different level, and students start to think about what asking for and listening to patients' stories can do for the caregiving relationship.

What unspoken stories can they observe when they go into a patient's room? Is anyone else there—a family member, a friend? Are there cards, photographs? Do they see any books or magazines, and, if so, which ones? Are there bits of food around, and, if so, what? Healthy snacks or junk food? Is the patient listening to music, and, if so, is it classical, jazz, country, or heavy metal?

What can all these little details tell them about the person in the bed? By paying attention and taking cues from the environment, medical students are engaging in eye and ear training for what is to be learned beyond the patient's "principle complaint" and typical charted information. They learn that each clinical case is embodied in a real person who lives his or her particular story in a totally unique fashion.

From noticing, the students move on to asking questions. If they see a photograph on a patient's nightstand, they say, "Tell me who's in your picture." Showing interest in the whole person is an act of shared humanity. A simple question is an invitation to tell a story, and they discover that little details are the doorways to larger stories and to building relationships.

Linda explains:

The world of patients and families is frightening territory, often rooted in fear of the unknown and loss of meaning, independence, and integrity. Recounting the events of an illness or injury in a story eases these feelings and is often the beginning of healing.

Susan Sontag once said that when you are ill, it's like being in a foreign kingdom. Asking for stories is a bridge back from exile, a place of refuge when all else feels strange, and an important route to insight, compassion, empathy, connection, community. Joan Didion said, "We tell ourselves stories to live."

Health care professionals, too, have stories to tell. These men and women keep company with the suffering of others and walk with them through profound events. The world of health care professionals is full of long hours, pressured situations, hard work, miracles, and tragedies. It can be a raw place with its own pain, fear of the unknown, and loss of meaning. For health care professionals, too, then, telling their stories helps provide comfort and healing for the dramatic work they do. For all, telling stories helps provide meaning in chaos.

It Doesn't Take Much

I'm a third-year medical student, a position that grants me the title of "clerk," and I have just finished my first three-month rotation. The word in med school is that your clerkship year is a year of feeling dumb. You're working in hospitals and clinics, and you're wearing a white coat, and people think you're a real doctor. Even with two years of medical school under your belt, though, all you can think about is how huge and vast is the knowledge you don't yet have!

As humbling as this is, the good news is that, in these first three months, I've learned that although I may not feel smart, I can still contribute to someone's care. I can, with my words and actions, reassure people, provide comfort and support, and listen and not judge. I can make someone's scary time not so scary. While the real professionals are making the big decisions, I have learned that I'm not worthless. I have qualities and abilities that can genuinely help people. It doesn't take much.

For example, just last week, a thirty-five-year-old woman was in the gynecology clinic for a colposcopy. She'd had precancerous lesions on her cervix, and this procedure would remove them. It was my first day in this clinic and everything was new. For the doctor, though, this was going to be his seventeenth procedure of the day—something that would be performed quickly, taking only fifteen minutes.

The patient had her legs up in the air, supported by footrests—the most vulnerable position in the world for a woman. The doctor started the procedure. He is a nice man, but he is "efficient" and doesn't say much as he goes about his work. Sensing this woman's fear and her discomfort, I did what I could to help, squeezing her hand in encouragement and saying things like, "You're doing great" and "You're almost done."

I ran into this woman when she was leaving the clinic. She said, "I'm so glad you were with me. I know the doctor is an excellent surgeon, but his manner terrifies me. Your being there made it so much less awful."

Another woman was referred to the gynecology clinic for an investigation of persistent, heavy bleeding. She had refused a pelvic examination by her own family doctor, a male, and had waited a potentially life-threatening two years in order to see the female gynecologist of the clinic. Upon reading this information in the referral note, the female doctor was enraged that the referral had been made on the basis of gender. During her first introduction to this patient, she sternly explained that the patient was attending a teaching clinic where the students could very well be male, and she would have to allow their participation, regardless of gender, if she wanted to be seen.

Fortunately, for the patient, I was the student that day—a female. After I had taken her history, but before the examination, I presented her case to the doctor, in private. I mentioned that the woman was taking antidepressants and realized I had not determined the reason for this. The doctor asked me to get more information.

When I went back in to see the patient, she was lying on the examining table. I gently explained that I had forgotten to ask her why she was taking antidepressants. She completely broke down and started sobbing. The worry over her gynecological condition was not this patient's only source of stress. She revealed that she was going through a divorce and was not coping well. Trembling in the examination room, she seemed so sad and fragile. I covered her with a blanket, sat her up, and did what I could to soothe her. I asked her questions about her children, which calmed her and seemed to strengthen her spirits.

I reported all this to the doctor. When she came in to do the exam, she was not as brusque as she had been before. I continued to hold the woman's hand through the rest of the consult. She was so scared. There was so much going on in her life that she couldn't control.

I spoke to the senior resident about this patient later in the day. She said to me, "You were more of a doctor today than you've ever been. We can have a profound impact on people and can relieve so much suffering with communication and compassion."

On another day, a thirty-two-year-old woman and her husband came in because she was having a miscarriage and needed medical help. Even though miscarriages are relatively common, occurring in approximately 40 percent of medically detectable pregnancies within the first trimester (twelve weeks), this couple had been celebrating their first pregnancy, and they were devastated that it was ending. The attending physician actually asked me to stand by the woman's head to comfort her. I felt the doctor was appreciating that I could play an important role in the care of this couple. He sensed that his knowledge and skill weren't all that was needed in this situation—that empathy was important, too. With some doctors, I feel as though they and I have very different agendas; this day, I felt we were on the same page.

I'm learning so much this year. Of course, I'm learning lots about medical science and treatment techniques, but I'm also learning that the doctors I appreciate the most are those who know an enormous amount but who still take the time to explain things, in simple language, to their patients. I've observed that two different doctors can spend the same period of twelve minutes with a patient, but one patient will feel like it's been thirty minutes and the other will feel like everything is rushed.

It's such an art to validate someone's concerns, to listen, to ask questions, and to make the patient feel like he or she is playing an important role in the interaction. Words and body language are so important when people are feeling vulnerable.

It's an incredible privilege to be part of someone's health care and their well-being. I'm so grateful I can play a role. People look at you in a white coat, and you become "the trusted one." It's an amazing responsibility and one that I take very seriously. As a clerk, I may often feel dumb with regard to my medical knowledge, but I can be "smart" with regard to compassion. It doesn't take much, but it often makes all the difference in the world.

The White Coat

Every early morning, the surgeons, trailing a gaggle of medical students, clerks, and residents, make their rounds through the intensive care unit (ICU). The group travels from patient to patient—beds full of them. I could easily picture Mark in that herd. He was tall and graceful and, no doubt, fresh and bright even in the early morning: neat white coat, stethoscope nestled in the pocket, notebook and pen at the ready. Ambitious, smart, compassionate, and heartful. Every early morning.

A few days into his ICU rotation, Mark noticed that the group always passed by one patient, a woman in the corner bed. He began to wonder why she was never included in rounds, and it started to bother him. So one afternoon, when the unit was quiet, Mark found the time to go to check on her. He was allowed to do that, with the white coat and the look of authority he was just then learning to wear comfortably. He found her mostly still, heavily drugged against pain. Standing quietly at the foot of her bed, he reviewed her chart: a tumor, growing deep in her brain, was killing her.

Sitting in my office a few days later, Mark told me about it. The two of us had made an arrangement some months before when Mark had first come by to talk about issues concerning informed consent. One of my roles in the clinical ethics service was to help students like him work through difficult issues they were learning to face as they became doctors. Since that time, he had come by the office every once in a while to tell me stories from his practice. It seemed to help him to talk about things, and it certainly helped me to gain some understanding of the evolution of a medical practitioner. Snapshots.

And now this.

After reviewing the woman's chart, Mark had spoken with one of the nurses who was looking after the patient.

"She'll die soon," the nurse told him. "Shame she'll die alone."

In my office, the young man stretched out his long legs and looked out the window behind me. He fiddled with the name tag pinned to his white coat, folded neatly in his lap.

"The patient is undocumented," he explained. "No papers that they could find. No health coverage. No status." A pause. "And alone."

I know this happens, even in Canada, once in a while—people fall through the cracks, especially if they have no home, no address. Or if they land here illegally. Sometimes they don't know how to get health insurance. Even here.

"Well," Mark continued, "she gets good care and everything. It's just that there isn't anyone there to pay"—he paused, searching for the right word—"particular attention to her. No one there just for her."

He fell silent for a moment.

"So I decided I'd try to find out if there was anyone around for her. You know, family or friends. Just someone who isn't wearing one of these." He touched the white coat in his lap.

"Wow," I nodded. "That's great."

Mark didn't look happy, though—no smile.

He gave a small shrug. "Well, it took me awhile, but I did track down a sister."

"Great."

He looked out the window at the darkening sky; the sun sets early in the late autumn.

"Yeah, well turns out the sister lives in Montreal. Used to live in a car but got some help and found a room. Yeah—a room. So she's poor, too."

"What did you do?"

"I tracked her down and called her to tell her that her sister's sick and that she should find a way to come here as soon as possible."

Mark traced the letters engraved into the plastic of his name tag, running his fingers over the black lines.

"Is she coming?"

"Yeah, at least I think she is. She said she'd take the bus down. Should be here by tomorrow."

Still no smile.

"So why aren't you happy?"

Mark straightened up, smoothed the white coat, and looked at me again.

"This morning I reported the news to my supervisor. I told him that I had tracked down the sister so that the patient won't have to die alone. I was proud of myself and thought he'd be happy, too."

"And? What did he say?"

"He wasn't happy with me, that's for sure. He told me that it isn't my job to hold hands with patients, and that if I wanted to do any more of that, I should go and be a social worker. Or a nurse."

Damn, I thought, a familiar seed of disappointment beginning to take root.

"And he told me I'd lose my place in the program if I ever did that again."

Damn again.

"I can't afford to lose my spot," Mark went on. "I can't take that risk."

His hands lay flat and still on top of the white coat.

"Of course not," I answered. "Of course not. You shouldn't risk it."

The sound of traffic from outside seeped into the room, now full of shadows.

Mark stood up, shifting the white coat to the table beside him. I stood up and faced him—his green eyes were clear and direct.

"So, I've made a decision," he said. "I'm going to take off my values." He mimed taking off a coat. "And I'm going to pack them into a box." He acted out folding an imaginary coat and putting it into a box.

"And put that box up on a shelf for the duration of my training."

He reached up and placed the box on a high shelf, putting his values in storage. He brushed his hands together, in a "so that's that" gesture, and turned back to me. He half-smiled, then shrugged.

"I only hope they'll still be there when I can come back for them."

I nodded. "I have no doubt—absolutely no doubt."

Mark gathered up his things. I walked him to the door of my office and opened it onto the empty hallway. We shook hands and thanked each other. I watched him walk away. He paused at the heavy blue metal door and turned to offer a small wave good-bye. I waved in reply and went back inside my office, pulling the door closed behind me. I stood there for a couple of minutes, gathering the bits of my day, trying to stitch them together around the hole left behind by Mark's story. It felt like a battle on the verge of being lost.

◆ ◆ ◆

When things slow with the coming of summer, the hospital staff members grab time for coffee and head outside for some air. The best seats are the ones under the trees.

This particular hot afternoon, a nurse I know well is sitting across from me, beaming from ear to ear, her coffee barely touched. She has worked at this hospital for decades. She's one of the pillars of the place.

She's been telling me a story of a new resident on her service—what a great guy he is, how stubbornly he stands up for what he knows is right.

"He says he knows you," she tells me.

"Yeah? What's his name?"

"Mark," she answers. "He's pretty great."

It's been three years since I've seen Mark—three years since I've given his box of values much thought. Time flows too full and too fast.

"He's like a dog with a bone," she continues. "I've seen him stand up for patients over and over again."

I think back to the woman in the ICU. I wonder if her sister ever arrived to be with her when she died. Three years ago.

"He saved a patient's life last week." The nurse goes on, "He pushed and pushed to be sure that a test was done when the senior guys thought it wasn't necessary. Saved the guy's life." She smiles again. "It really is great to see that in such a young doc."

I smile. "It certainly is." A streetcar rumbles past. "I never doubted that he'd be that good. Never once."

Battle won. Score one for the good guys.

· · · · ·

Linda Clarke is a writer and storyteller and works with members of the health care community, including medical students, to help them see the power of story in how they understand themselves, patients, families, and other caregivers. In her years in health care, Linda has been part of many privileged encounters. One of them is the seed of this story.

When the World Turns Upside Down: A Doctor Experiences Being a Patient

I remember going to a lecture in early June, a couple of weeks before my family practice residency was to end. I have always had excellent vision, and so, even though I had been up all night, I was surprised that I couldn't read the notes on the screen. *Something's not right,* I thought, but my mind quickly talked itself out of worrying, talking back to itself with, *I must have strained my eyes from reading so much and working so hard.*

A week later, I had to admit I couldn't read my patients' monitors, and so I made an appointment to get glasses. The eye doctor didn't ask me if I had any other troubling symptoms, probably presuming that because I am a doctor I would have checked out any other possible causes for my impaired vision.

In the next days and weeks, I also experienced weight loss, excessive thirst, and frequent urination. I remember drinking huge amounts of water and having to go to the bathroom between every patient. I noted that a pair of pants I had bought in May were falling off of me in June. Despite all of the clues, I avoided facing reality. Of course, if I had been one of my patients, I would have diagnosed myself in a minute.

At some point, the thought did cross my mind that perhaps I had diabetes, but then I argued to myself, *It can't possibly be true. I'm just worried and magnifying everything, just like I did all through med school, thinking I had every disease in the book.*

My boyfriend, also a doctor, said, "If you're really worried, why don't you test yourself at work?" But I didn't. It was a good idea, of course, but somewhere in my head there was a voice saying, *I don't have time for this, and anyway, doctors aren't supposed to get sick!* Looking back, I can see that deep, deep down, I was afraid.

Instead of addressing my fears, I did what I usually do—I carried on. My residency ended in late June. As a treat to myself, I visited my grandmother in Florida for a week. While I was visiting her, I stood on some scales and discovered I had lost twelve pounds in two months. I decided I'd have to make an appointment with my clinic when I returned home.

At the doctor's office, I saw my physician's assistant. I must have glossed over or selectively shared some of what had been happening because she didn't immediately say, "You have diabetes." Neither did she even do the obvious, like checking my blood or urine, which could have been done right there in the office. Instead, we started thinking about other things that might have caused some of my symptoms. Stress? Tuberculosis? A parasite?

I left the clinic having had blood drawn, which would be sent to a lab, and wearing a tuberculosis patch test. Both tests would give results in forty-eight hours. I went to my boyfriend's and just sat and sobbed. I knew something was terribly wrong.

I had been to the clinic on a Wednesday. By Friday, I was preparing to drive to Washington to write an all-day exam on Saturday. This exam was a big deal. You have to sign up for it a year in advance, the fee is about $1,000, and you have to pass it to be board certified as a family practice physician. Annette, a doctor and also a friend who would be writing the same exam, came over to my apartment. We were going to travel to Washington together. I told her I had to call the clinic for some test results before we left.

I reached the office nurse and told her that the tuberculosis test was negative and asked her if the results were in from the blood lab. She started to read them to me. "Well, you're not anemic; your thyroid is fine; your blood sugar is 300. Wow! What did you eat?" I calmly said, "Oh, yeah! That's too high." And I hung up.

As a doctor, I understood that normal blood sugar levels are supposed to be between 70 and 120, and mine were 300. My mind was racing. All I could think was, *Can I pretend not to have this information until after the exam? How do I get myself to Washington?* Oddly enough, even though tears were streaming down my face, I actually felt a bit of relief. At least now I knew what I was dealing with. I quickly leapt into problem-solving mode.

I turned to Annette and blurted out, "I have diabetes! I know I have to deal with this, but I've got to keep going until tomorrow night."

Meanwhile, my physician's assistant was desperately trying to reach me, frantic that I'd been given my results over the phone. I was asked to come into the clinic right away. The standard procedure for a person newly diagnosed with Type 1 diabetes is to be admitted to the hospital for intravenous administration of fluids and insulin and for education. Quite predictably, I rejected that option, saying, "But I already know how to do all that stuff, and I've got to write an exam tomorrow!"

Even though I was emotionally seesawing—crying one minute and laughing the next—my attitude was, "Give me the fast course—let's get going!" On the checklist for stages of grief, I'd already done denial and didn't have time for anger. I was negotiating and was ready for action.

My clinic agreed to try to work with my determination level. They set me up on an IV in a little office at the back of the clinic where I had access to a phone to be able to call family and friends. The nurse showed me how to measure and inject insulin and talked to me about my diet. In a matter of hours, I felt I had the tools I needed for the weekend. Annette and I were on the road, heading toward Washington. I was postponing dealing with the rest of my life until Monday.

Washington is my home, and so Annette and I had dinner with my parents. It was comforting to be there and to be able to talk things out. Even though Annette and I actually know quite a bit about diabetes, the scene after dinner looked like an elementary science class. Here were two doctors and my mother, a nurse, all trying to figure out how to read the numbers on a syringe and do an insulin injection. I caught myself thinking, *We are trained professionals who are supposed to know how to do this. I can't imagine how enormously difficult and stressful this must be for people who can't read or who are afraid of needles!*

I barely remember the exam. Getting meals and safely giving myself the appropriate amount of insulin consumed my mind. When I returned home after the weekend, I turned my house into "diabetes camp." Friends ate dinner with me every night, to be supportive and to learn my dietary changes with me. I read numerous books about diabetes. I went to the grocery store and read labels. I threw out "bad" stuff like six boxes of brown sugar I had in my cupboard and tried every kind of artificial sugar going. Most importantly, my blood sugar returned to normal.

I also took the time to see a doctor who specializes in diabetes. She was wonderful and somehow had the perfect balance of treating me with respect for my medical knowledge while also being very clear that I was a patient. Because this was her field, she was able to share with me some of the hopeful developments in the world of diabetes.

"You'll be just fine," she reassured me, but she also said, in a very supportive way, "You don't have to do this all by yourself just because you are a doctor! In fact, I highly recommend you see a psychologist at least once. This is a really big thing in your life, and it might help to have someone to talk to." She was right.

The psychologist helped me surface feelings of guilt I had about somehow personally causing this disease. The sessions also provided a forum for working through some decisions I've had to make in terms of my career.

Having diabetes has forced me to make sure my priorities are right. For example, even though I trained for three years to deliver babies and am good at it, I've chosen not to include that in my practice. Irregular sleeping and eating makes it much more difficult to control my blood sugar levels.

The last year and a half has been an amazing journey for me. I've had to make the transition from being a person with nothing wrong with my body to a person with diabetes. In the process, I've learned that when you have a chronic illness like diabetes, you don't get to take a vacation from it. It's never going to go away, and it's hard work. In spite of being used to being in control of my world, I'm also learning that diabetes is a beast that you can't always control no matter how particular you are about management.

I've been so fortunate all my life. I've had lots of support and resources to pursue my dreams, and I've been good at what I've done. Now I'm trying to come to terms with things I can't do. Or, more accurately phrased, I'm trying to learn that just because I can do everything, I don't have to!

I'm slowly coming to accept that I'm a human being with some limitations. I've been criticized in the past for not taking very much time for myself. Now, I'm trying to do that and to feel comfortable with it. It's humbling!

It's also humbling to realize, until now, how little I really understood about people's daily lives. I used to think I was very aware of and sympathetic to the difficulties my patients faced. Now, though, I have a new awareness and new appreciation for the fact that lots of people are silently, privately dealing with a wide array of challenges. My level of understanding for how complex life can be, on a day-to-day basis, has become much deeper.

Although I wouldn't wish a chronic disease on anyone, I am starting to see the positive impact diabetes has had on how I approach life and on how I approach being a doctor. I am gentler toward patients who have put off coming to see me, who have tried to pretend that whatever they have will go away. I also am more appreciative of the important, supportive, and useful role psychologists and counselors can play. Most profoundly, I think I now better understand the word *empathy*.

· · · · ·

This doctor went on to get a graduate degree in public health. She is now the lead physician in a community health center. She and her boyfriend referred to in this story got married and now have 2 young children.

The Other Side of the Bed

Last week life smacked me in the face with a deeper understanding of the "patient and family experience."

The usual clinical summary of my "case" would read something like this:

> This sixty-two-year-old male noticed the sudden onset
> of imbalance while browsing in front of the refrigerator.
> Despite being a physician and knowing better (okay, my
> self-critical commentary here), instead of first calling 911,
> he asked his brother to drive him to Methodist Hospital.
> On arrival he displayed staggering gait, inability to tan-
> dem walk, and perhaps mildly slurred speech. A code 99
> (possible stroke) was called. CT scan of the brain and a
> cerebral magnetic resonance angiogram (MRA) did not
> show an acute cerebral hemorrhage or infarct (stroke).
> The symptoms improved greatly during the first three
> hours and completely resolved within twelve hours. He
> was discharged to home on low-dose aspirin therapy for
> presumptive diagnosis of transient ischemic attack (TIA).

Notice the way a clinical summary eliminates how the patient and family experience the events. These summaries present essential short-hand to communicate clinical meaning, but necessarily omit relating the experience through the perspective of the patient and family.

What Did I Experience from the Other Side of the Bed?

My background remains different than most patients who are hospitalized at Methodist. I have spent nearly every working day of the last twenty years at Methodist. Methodist feels warm and familiar. Additionally, I have years of training and experience as a physician.

This training allowed me to immediately attribute the sudden balance problem to specific blood vessels serving the brain. As I lay on the floor, alone at home (my wife and daughter were dropping off flowers at the Peter Hobart Memorial site for the school children who died on a field trip in St. Paul), I briefly entertained "toughing it out" on my own, knowing that if it was a TIA, I would be better soon and could start aspirin therapy. Looking back, I could frame this as an utterly stupid approach or, more respectfully, recognize my thinking for what it was—the patient experience of denial.

Once I arrived at the Methodist emergency department, a code was called. Code 99 for a possible stroke entails an elegantly choreographed and standardized dance of simultaneous evaluation and treatment. These codes save brains and lives. From the other side of the bed, I experienced the code 99 as a hazy throng surrounding and touching me—simultaneously removing my shirt, starting an IV, placing electrodes, drawing blood, performing vitals, checking my oxygen level, doing an electrocardiogram, sticking my finger for a blood sugar, asking me questions, showing me pictures to describe, requesting me to read several sentences, instructing me to wrinkle my eyebrows, move my eyes, stick out my tongue, shrug my shoulders, and lift my limbs. I was scared *before* the code 99; the emergency activities increased my fear.

Minutes later, the ceiling became a moving blur as I was wheeled to radiology for a CT scan. (I had never considered moving ceilings as part of the patient experience, but when else do we lie on our backs, gazing up at ceilings as transporters navigate carts through halls and elevators?)

I started to transfer myself from the cart to the X-ray table, but was immediately told that the team would put a transfer board under me, and all I needed to do was cross my hands over my chest. I knew I was capable of transferring on my own, but I had entered the strange and foreign land in my beloved hospital. The team was appropriately following a transfer protocol to keep me safe.

Back in the emergency department, a neurologist explained the findings of the CT scan and discussed the benefits versus the risks of "lytic therapy." When I practiced as a physician, I excelled in understanding evidence-based medicine, the science of clinical decision making, as well as the art of decision making in the face of uncertainty, unknowns, and unknowables. On the other side of the bed, however, I simply basked in the warm glow of Ativan and trust in the doctor. I could not navigate the foreign territory of decision making. Fortunately, my brother, an ER physician, discussed options with my doctor and, together, they worked out a plan. I was admitted for observation and additional tests. I went home the next day feeling fine, though changed.

What I experienced was frightening and foreign, despite my familiarity with hospitals and medicine. Imagine how patients and families feel who do not bring a medical background to their experiences.

How I Felt Supported

Although my experience was sobering, I felt wonderfully supported throughout my hospital stay. Everyone I interacted with— physicians, nurses, nursing aides, transporters, volunteers, individuals working in the echocardiography lab, radiology, the flying squad, those in environmental and food services—combined an air of professional competency with warm compassion and empathy.

I sensed that the care was centered on me as the patient. I felt secure and confident in my care as I watched individuals from different areas assist one another. For example, the nurses on the sixth floor gladly provided an extra pair of helping hands to the individual performing the echocardiogram.

I received constant updates about what to expect, and people routinely asked me whether I needed anything. And perhaps most importantly, within the limits of being safely tethered to a bed that sounded an alarm if I tried to get up on my own, I was given choices. Even small choices, such as the ability to select foods from the room service menu and to choose who in the family I wanted updated, acted as an antidote to my sense of vulnerability.

The Essence of the Patient and Family Experience

The patient and family experience is not about "definitely recommend" scores, even though that is our best proxy measure. It is not about scripts, though they can be helpful. It is not about better business—it is the core of our business. It is not about pleasing patients and families, though it begins with a sense of serving.

It is about how we as human beings support our fellow human beings during scary, uncertain, and foreign times. It is about healing relationships for patients and families, and, at times, for healers. It is about seeing the world through the eyes of those we serve and helping to make that world less foreboding and foreign. It is about understanding the stories of patients and, with them, changing their stories as we compose our own.

We all take our turns on the "other side of the bed." I was fortunate that after my time spent in that strange and foreign land, I am fine. We may not all have the same outcomes, but we all desire and deserve the same great experience.

When I tap into my experiences as a patient, our Park Nicollet vision comes alive: "Everyone caring, every day, creating, with the individuals we serve, optimal health and greater value."

I would enjoy hearing your experiences as patients and how those experiences influence your approach to the patient in front of you. Given that you may also become a patient, what does our vision statement mean to you?

· · · · ·

Some excellent medical writing can be found in the blogs of health care leaders. This story is one selection from the blog of Dr. David Abelson, senior executive vice president of Health Partners and chief executive officer of Park Nicollet Health Services in Minneapolis. He says, "I started an internal blog several years ago, which is read widely by staff. This blog has helped to create conversations about patient- and family-centered care in our institution and beyond. I sometimes use my own health care experiences to enhance the conversations." The full blog can be found at http://drabelsonconnects.tumblr.com/.

Behind a Locked Door

This is our story as I remember it.

One day I came home from work, and my husband was confused. In all the years we'd been married, I'd never known him to be confused. He was sitting in the family room, and he looked frightened.

I said, "Bill, what's going on?" He said, "Well, I was just going to get up and go look outside for Joey." I said, "Bill, Joey's not here." He insisted, "Oh yes, we just came back from vacation. Joey just went outside, and I was going to check on him."

I was alarmed and said, "Bill, I think you're a little confused. I'm concerned because this morning you told me you had a headache. Maybe we should go to the hospital." He resisted, but I simply told him, "Bill, if something was to happen to you, I might be held responsible because I didn't do what was in your best interest. We can come home if everything is okay."

And so we went to the emergency room, where we learned that my husband had a small bleed in his brain. We were told that we needed to go to another hospital that had a neurosurgeon on staff. My husband was transported by ambulance to a hospital about a mile away, and I followed him there in our car.

I want to stop here and tell you a bit about my husband and about myself. My name is Jackie Gruzenski, and I am a nurse involved in the field of psychiatric nursing. My husband's name was Dr. William Gruzenski. He was a psychiatrist for forty years, and he was a chief medical officer for the last twelve years of his career.

Bill was a very good doctor and a very good husband. And toward the end of his life, he realized that all of his degrees, along with money and material possessions, didn't matter. They were nothing. He just wanted to have me with him. We loved each other very deeply, and we wanted to share our last days and moments together, but I'm getting ahead of myself.

When we got to the second hospital, my husband was in the emergency room from about 7:00 p.m. until about 6:00 a.m. the next morning. At some point, he started to develop a hypertensive crisis, and the staff could not bring his blood pressure down. They started an IV medication, which required that he be monitored closely in the intensive care unit (ICU).

Of course, I went with him as he was transferred from emergency to ICU. When we got to the ICU door, I was told, "Now, just go into the waiting room. We're going to settle your husband, and then we'll come and get you."

I was a nervous wreck while I waited. I knew my husband had been pretty sick while in emergency. What if he got more confused? What if he lost even this current level of functioning and wouldn't remember me? The longer I waited, the more my anxiety grew.

The waiting room was a small area, with chairs around the perimeter, except by the locked door. After an hour with no news, I saw a phone on the wall and called. I said to the voice on the other end, "My name is Mrs. Gruzenski. I was informed that my husband was going to be settled and that someone would come and get me."

The next thing I knew a young, perky nurse came out, greeted me, and then directed me totally away from my husband, away from the door to the ICU, to a little room. She proceeded to give me the strict policies and procedures for the ICU, including that visitation was allowed only four times a day for thirty minutes each time.

Not believing what I was hearing, I said, "But my husband is going to be worried that I am not with him. We are the center of each other's lives—we are only apart when we are at work!" Her response was, "Well, you can't be with him. Those are the rules."

I lived ten miles away. What was I supposed to do between these widely spaced thirty-minute visits? I felt I had to play by the rules. I was afraid that if I questioned too much or was abrupt with someone, they would treat my husband meanly. And because he was behind a locked door, I would never know.

I didn't know what else to do and so, shortly before 8:00 a.m., I went home to get some rest. Ironically, just after I got home and started to settle after our long night in the ER, I got a flurry of calls from different residents who wanted information about my husband. They never said, "Come over and visit. He's missing you." They called because they needed the information I could give them, but they kept me locked out.

When I was able to have my first visit the next day, my husband asked where I had been. I explained that there were very limited visiting hours. This prompted my husband to speak to his nurse and say, "You know, she's not a visitor. She's my wife!" But he was informed that didn't matter, that there were rules, and that I was a visitor and had to be treated as a visitor.

The rule trumped both of us and what we wanted. The rule meant he had to suffer alone. This was an accredited hospital, but in my view it was archaic. Staff hid behind the rules rather than using their heads and their hearts.

Over the next few days, I saw that my not being there with my husband was leading to more and more distress for him. As he became more ill, he would not allow the nurses to wash him, and he would not eat their food. He was doing everything he could do to get the staff's attention to revisit the visiting restrictions. If I'd been allowed to stay, I'm sure I could have helped with feeding, with bathing, and with toileting. I'm certain I could have calmed him and helped lower his blood pressure.

I was treated as though I was an enemy, but all I wanted was to be with him, to share the last days of his life. I had always been his anchor. I was the person who navigated the everyday waters of his life. The hospital's rules meant that he was adrift, and I was lost.

During his hospitalization, he was not afforded the respect he had given to all his patients and the nurses and doctors he had worked with each day. For example, the ICU staff never asked him how he would like to be addressed. They called him "Bill" when he should have been addressed as "Doctor Gruzenski." He wouldn't have thought of calling a resident by his first name, and there were only a few people in his life, his inner circle of family and friends, who called him "Bill."

One day, I actually witnessed one doctor refer to my husband not even as "Bill" but as "Billy." I followed this doctor out of the ICU and challenged him saying "Would you think you were valued as a medical professional, and that your life had meant something if, in forty years' time, someone called you 'Billy'? 'Billy' is what you call some young boy you like, not someone who is sixty-eight years old and is a dignified gentleman and physician."

My husband earned the title of "Doctor." He attended four years of medical school, one year of internship, four years as a resident psychiatrist, and he was board certified in psychiatry. He had earned respect by exceeding all the societal standards for being addressed as "Doctor." These achievements should not be washed away once you are hospitalized. In fact, I believe my husband might have felt a little safer if he had been addressed as "Doctor."

My husband was in the ICU for eight of the last sixteen days of his life, and there were lots of missed opportunities for us. He wanted me there more than I was allowed. We missed time together we could have had. I feel it was a very cruel thing that was done to us.

We both knew the gravity of his condition, and my husband wanted quality of life, not quantity. I was a large part of the quality he wanted, but I was locked out for the greater part of his last days.

After my husband died, I felt I had to do something so that what happened to us wouldn't happen to anyone else. I wrote letters to the chief executive officer of the hospital. I wrote to the chief of the medical staff. I wrote to the chief of nursing. And I wrote to the chaplain. The only person I ever heard from was the chaplain. No one apologized or said they would change the rules.

I believe more harm comes when family are not actively involved, and research is proving my belief is sound. And so I will continue to tell my story. I hope that if I tell it enough times, maybe people who write the rules in hospitals will realize that loved ones are advocates, not visitors.

I will never stop advocating for the elimination of visiting hours.

· · · · ·

Jackie Gruzenski's story inspired the 2014 launching of Better Together: Partnering with Families, an international campaign led by the Institute for Patient- and Family-Centered Care to forever change the concept of families as visitors. Go to www.ipfcc.org/bettertogether/ for further information. This family's story was also shared by Don Berwick in his address to the Yale School of Medicine graduating class in 2010, inspiring the next generation of physicians to respect the preferences, choices, priorities, and values of patients and families, and no longer to label families as visitors in hospital settings.

Creating a Culture

I first became a parent in the late 1980s. Like so many first-time parents, I read everything I could and was highly motivated to be the best parent possible. While pregnant, I stayed away from microwaves; I watched what I ate; I asked questions of my obstetrician; and I was prepared to advocate for my children and to protect them from harm. I felt empowered and confident.

Yet for all my good intentions and diligence, I felt completely unprepared, in 1991, when I learned our second-born son had a life-threatening chronic illness. Standing in a crowded hallway of The Children's Hospital of Philadelphia (CHOP), my husband and I learned that our baby William had cystic fibrosis (CF). As the doctor gave us the details about our son's illness, I remember wanting to find a quiet place to sit down. My knees were buckling, and my only option was to lean against the wall. As the doctor continued, I was distracted by a constantly ringing telephone. I kept wishing someone would answer it so I could focus on what the doctor was saying.

As the doctor described the impact CF would have on our little boy, I saw my husband's eyes well with tears. I ached inside thinking, *We have been married for five years and I have never seen him cry.* I desperately wanted to find a private place where we could be together and support each other. I knew it wasn't that this good doctor didn't know better or had neglected to find a more comforting location to share this news. It was just that, at the time, there simply was no physical space to share this kind of news privately. No alternatives existed for staff or families.

From the early days of learning about CF, I felt so isolated. I felt no one, not even our family and friends, knew what it was like to be me at that moment. Even when I was living at the hospital, with people all around me, I felt alone. I had so many more questions than answers. For all I had read before my pregnancies, I now had no road map for how to be the mom of a chronically ill baby.

I lacked the confidence I had had as a new mom. I now felt uncertain; therapeutic decisions seemed unclear; and the medical terms and jargon were confusing. I didn't know how I would fit all these new medicines, doctor appointments, hospital visits, and therapies into our "normal" life. I had no context in my personal life for living with chronic illness. I was used to solving problems, and I was desperately struggling to figure out how I was going to fix this.

On our third night in the hospital, I was sitting beside our son's crib, still trying to comprehend what all this would mean for him and for our family. A nurse came in to the room and quietly said, "Mrs. Schlucter, a mom and her daughter were admitted last night. Her daughter has been living with CF for twelve years. If you want, I can introduce you."

Later that night, down the hall in the playroom, this other mom and I met. The nurse had ordered coffee for us. This was the first CF mom I had ever met, and she became my lifeline to this new world. She had the answers to so many questions that only another mom raising a child with CF could answer. That night, that nurse did something so small yet so important. She recognized the reality that families often need the unique support that can come only from another parent.

I recall another small gesture in those early days. Our son's pulmonologist asked us if we would like to see what his team was looking at with respect to our son's lungs. "Come with me and I'll show you." It was such a privilege to walk beside this eminent physician to the clinician's radiology viewing room. He understood that we wanted to know everything we could about our son's condition, and we wanted to be included in the decisions about his care.

The actions of that nurse and that doctor stand out in my memory because, at that time, The Children's Hospital of Philadelphia (CHOP) had neither a culture nor an environment designed to support patients and families. These gestures, which honored my hope to be the best mother I could be of a sick little boy, were like beacons of what could be possible compared to what was more commonplace in existing medical models.

In 1992, we learned, before she was even born, that our daughter Julia would also have cystic fibrosis. CHOP became increasingly familiar and the opportunities to partner for change expanded.

When she was three, Julia needed a picc (peripherally inserted central catheter) line for her antibiotic therapy. Having been a patient in and out of the hospital by the age of three, Julia already knew well to cling tightly to me when nurses and doctors approached. As the nurse greeted us to walk to the conscious sedation unit, Julia squeezed me tighter and tighter. We were stopped at a door with a large stop sign that read ABSOLUTELY NO ONE BEYOND THIS POINT. I proceeded to go through the door with Julia because it didn't occur to me that I was "no one"—I was Julia's mother; I knew how to comfort her and keep her calm. Sadly, my logic did not prevail and, while Julia screamed desperately, the nurse literally peeled her off me and took her away. As they started Julia's procedure, I kept my ear pressed to the door because I needed to hear when she stopped screaming.

What was routine for staff was scarring for me. This was my first understanding of the sheer agony of being separated from my child. I believed there must be approaches to these moments that helped families stay as united with their children as possible and be included in the decision and preparation when separation was the only option.

I now understood just how broken a mother's heart could be. I believed that what I was experiencing was unique to pediatrics, unique to the experience between a mother and her child. And then, everything changed with a phone call.

Across town, my father had suffered a heart attack and had been admitted to the intensive care unit (ICU) of an academic medical center. We are a large and loving family, and we gathered quickly. My mother was devoted to her husband. She had never been away from him for forty-six years; each one of his five children loved him dearly. We all wanted to be with him, but the rules were that only two people were allowed to visit, for fifteen minutes, once every two hours. And so we took turns. We sent in messages with those who were allowed in, past the locked doors. We all waited together for the hour and three-quarters, the 105 minutes, until another two of us could visit him again for fifteen minutes.

Tragically, it was during one of those periods of time when the rules of the intensive care unit dictated that "absolutely no one" could be at their loved one's bedside that my father died. My mother was on the other side of the unit door, forbidden to enter. So, this great man, who had lived his life surrounded by family, died alone because it was the wrong fifteen minutes.

I'll never forget my mother sobbing, saying, "I've never left him before, and when he needed me to be with him the most, I let him down." In that moment, I realized that what I'd thought was exclusive to the experience in pediatrics, of a mother not wanting to be separated from her child, was a universal experience. I now knew, all too well, that this human need to stay with your loved one at such a vulnerable time is true for everyone, every age, every place, every time.

Coincidentally, while William and Julia were still very young, The Children's Hospital of Philadelphia leadership team was setting the foundation to transform a world-class *medically* centered hospital to a world-class *family*-centered hospital. The hospital was looking for input from families about how it could improve the experience of care, so I wrote a letter to CHOP's chief executive officer.

I simply described a day in the life of my family at the hospital. It wasn't all negative, but I did describe what it was like to hear devastating news in a public place; what it felt like to sit for prolonged periods of time in a busy waiting room when your child is ill; how heart-wrenching it was for William's five-year-old brother, who was not allowed to visit, and could only wave to his brother from the elevator; and the agony of not being able to stay with your child during procedures. My basic point was to ask how such a world-class hospital that provided such excellent clinical care could be missing so many other pieces that make up the care experience for patients and families.

Within days, I received a call from the senior vice president for patient care who asked if I would be willing to work with them to create change. The next thing I knew, I was sharing my story with an executive forum, which included the chief executive officer, the chief operating officer, and the senior vice president for patient care. As a group and as individuals, they were completely engaged. They connected emotionally. They were ready to respond and develop a blueprint for change.

In 1994, I found myself at the table at the beginning of a massive cultural change at CHOP. I was glad to be there, not only for my children, but for all the other children and families served by this outstanding hospital. Since that first meeting, I can say, unequivocally, that CHOP has totally and completely transformed itself and has exceeded every dream I had at the time. CHOP made family-centered care a priority. The hospital supported and sustained this commitment by integrating core concepts of collaboration, flexibility, support, and information for families into its programs and policies. The hospital didn't just change programs; it changed its culture. It changed from a rushed, busy medical institution to a culture that is nationally recognized for respecting and involving families as valued partners in the care of their children.

This fundamental change was possible because both the hospital leadership and families were prepared to collaborate. Without the vision and commitment of senior leadership and their trust in the process of involving families, the sweeping changes in policy, programs, environment, and culture would not have been possible.

I could already feel the beginnings of these changes in culture when Julia was six years old. A lobe of her lung collapsed in the middle of the night, and we jumped into the car to rush to the hospital. Our sons were in the back, my husband was driving, and Julia was in my arms. We arrived at emergency and a security guard met us. He didn't challenge us; he softly said, "Are you right-handed or left-handed?" He then slipped a clipboard under my right arm and said, "Walk with me. Let's get you signed in quickly so your daughter can be seen right away." That security guard had many choices that night, and he chose to meet me where I was and help me navigate the process. I felt supported and in the right place. I was able to take my first real breath since leaving the house.

The most profound proof of this cultural change occurred recently. Julia, at the time, was eighteen years old and had to have cranial-based surgery to remove polyps from the back of her sinuses. By then, she had discovered her passion as a singer and was a pursuing a career as a performer. As a result, this surgery was very delicate, and great care was required to protect her vocal cords.

On the day of surgery, my husband and I sat with Julia in the waiting area. She was approached and asked if she would want her parents present during anesthesia induction and in the recovery room. She said, "Yes," and so we walked together with the health care team through the doors that once read ABSOLUTELY NO ONE BEYOND THIS POINT.

The anesthesiologist shared options he had investigated to protect Julia's vocal cords, and he gave her choices to consider. In case you are wondering if you can hold your eighteen-year-old little girl in your lap before anesthesia and in recovery, the answer is, "Yes, you can!"

My greatest sorrow will always be that I can't change the fact that two of my children have cystic fibrosis. But my experience with The Children's Hospital of Philadelphia has shown me that I can contribute to other changes. I learned, whether in pediatrics or in adult health care, when hospital leaders and families share a vision for the care experience and collaborate with one another, anything is possible.

· · · · ·

Juliette Schlucter had the honor of cofounding the Family Faculty Program at CHOP in 1994. This program was designed to provide teaching forums for new employees, nurses, and medical students. She was one of five family leaders who were available to share their personal stories and experiences with hospital staff from biomedical engineering to trauma surgeons.

These forums provided not just opportunities for the family leaders to tell their stories, but also safe circumstances for staff to ask the kinds of basic questions they didn't feel comfortable asking at the bedside.

In 1995, Juliette became the hospital's first paid professional family consultant. Today, the Family Consultant Program has grown to several paid professional family leaders who meet with families, create programs, and bring patient and family voices to communications and patient care.

1996 saw the establishment of the Family Advisory Council, which works to inform senior administrators, clinical leaders, and hospital committees at the strategic planning level. In 1997, a Family Resource Center was opened, providing space for information, support, and other resources. In 1999, the Youth Advisory Council was formed, which recruits teenage patients who meet monthly to provide input to improve the hospital, socially and physically, for patients and families.

Now, in 2014, families are given the choice to be present with their child throughout the care experience, including procedures. Parents can sleep comfortably at their child's bedside; siblings can visit; parents make presentations at Grand Rounds; family consultants are part of the hospital's safety and quality and bio-ethics committees; and a parent co-chairs the hospital's task force on "The Ideal Hospital Experience."

Reflections

"Always be kind, for everyone is fighting a hard battle."
—*Plato*

"Cure sometimes, treat often, comfort always."
—*Hippocrates*

"Remember that everyone you meet is afraid of something, loves something and has lost something."
—*H. Jackson Brown Jr.*

Different Stories, Similar Echoes
To Fix, Help, or Serve
When One Is Overwhelmed
The Intensity of Memories
Moving On

Different Stories, Similar Echoes

Such diversity, yet such similarity. In spite of the fact that each and every story in *Privileged Presence* is unique, what is striking is the use of similar phrases and the repeated references to what matters. In the straightforward reading of these different stories, whether from the point of view of a patient, family member, or health care professional, it becomes clear, over and over again, that it is the simplest things that make huge differences.

From Florida to Ontario and California to Nova Scotia, patients, family members, and health care professionals shared their unique health care stories. Yet, from this great range of geography, gender, age, circumstance, and perspective, what has emerged can be compared to the many different voices that make up a choir. Like repeating melodies in a major choral work, consistent themes about what makes health care experiences positive echo and resonate throughout *Privileged Presence*, creating a sense of harmony even though the notes are different.

The echoes from the patient and family sections of the choir are simple and include the following:

- Understand that first impressions are important and can set me on a path of fear or hope.
- Acknowledge me . . . say "hello"; introduce yourself; find out who I am as a person and who we are as a family.
- Listen to me. I know what's normal and abnormal for me. I can help you figure out what's going on and what works and what doesn't work.
- Honor my family as partners in my care, especially if I can't speak for myself. Please listen to my family. They know me well, can be my advocates, and can help you, too.

- Look at me, beyond my words. I may not say everything that I am feeling, but I may show you what's inside. My body language may help you read my heart.

- Share information with me and my family members, and be honest. Feeling ignorant and isolated is so much worse than knowing the truth.

- Appreciate any initiatives I may have taken to access information from sources such as other patients and from the Internet.

- Take time to explain things and to ask if I/we have questions. If you help me/us understand and adjust, it will save time for all of us in the long run.

- See past what I have to who I am.

- Respect me for what I can do, not just for what is wrong with me.

- Ask me to consider treatment options and to be a partner in decision making.

- Coordinate and communicate what you are doing with others who are involved in my care.

- Encourage me to participate, as much as I choose and can, in my care and treatment. I want to be more involved than simply following directions.

- Invite me to use my strengths and to participate in my care and recovery.

- Consider what it will be like for me and my family when I go home. Help us plan, prepare, and know what to expect, as well as how to access help.

- Be flexible and bend or suspend rules when appropriate for my situation.

- Know that I enjoy knowing about you, too; it helps me feel connected to you as a partner in my care.

- Apologize. Say, "I'm sorry," and explain what happened if a mistake is made or if things don't go well.

These requests, or "invitations to provide good care," were cited directly or indirectly time and time again. Repeatedly, the stories in *Privileged Presence* show us how kindness, goodness, and common sense enrich health care relationships. They are simple acts of humanity and are neither complicated nor costly.

Many health care professionals intuitively understand how important it is to listen, to share information, to collaborate, to show respect, to take time, and to humbly pay attention. They know that the words they choose, the way they stand or sit, the interest they show, and the gestures of kindness they offer can make a difference to clinical outcomes and how patients and families manage their illnesses and feel about their care.

It is important to include these responsive elements of care in the training of future health care professionals. It is widely known that many medical students, for example, arrive with the values of compassion and collaboration, but that the older style of training extinguishes these values rather than support and develop them. Think of the young man in the story "The White Coat." He needed positive role models rather than threats.

The melodic notes that echo from the health care professional sections of the choir are well summed up in a quote of Mahatma Gandhi in which he was talking about "customers" but is equally relevant to a patient or a family member:

> *. . . He may be dependent on us. We are also dependent on him. He is not an interruption of our work. He is the purpose of it. He is not an outsider to our business. He is part of it. We are not doing him a favor by serving him. He is doing us a favor by giving us the opportunity to do so.*

To Fix, Help, or Serve

It is significant that Gandhi used the verb *serving*. In the world of health care, professionals spend years learning how to identify and to *fix* problems; their basic intention is to *help*. There are, however, profound differences among the verbs to *fix, help,* and *serve* from the patient's point of view.

Fixing stems from a judgment that the other person cannot do something, and the act of fixing takes away the potential for individuals to experience solving dilemmas for themselves. *Helping* usually occurs when someone stronger or smarter *assists*, which can result in the helper taking over and undermining the self-reliance of the person being helped. *Serving*, on the other hand, is the act of offering what is needed, what is appropriate, or what has been requested without assuming that the person making the request is annoying, incapable, or powerless.

Serving keeps the focus of control more on the person being served than on the server. When you fix, you see someone as broken, and when you help, you see someone as weak. When you serve, though, you see someone as whole. Serving is more likely to create a relationship of equals rather than one of hierarchy.

When One Is Overwhelmed

Ill health and injury can overwhelm even the smartest, strongest, and most vocal among us. Many patients and families who shared stories for this book were highly accomplished in their own day-to-day lives—business owners, elected politicians, lawyers, university professors. Some of them were even health care professionals.

And yet, many of them said they felt so completely vulnerable and intimidated by their health care encounters that they acted as though they had become paralyzed or mute. Comments such as "I didn't want to rock the boat" or "I didn't want to make the staff angry" came from a sense of fear that they would be ignored or that care would be withheld. A comment like "I was too stunned to speak" was made when someone felt so disregarded that he or she almost felt invisible. How do you speak if you feel you are not even seen?

In some cases, people took evasive action and voted with their feet. It was as though it felt safer and simpler to change health care providers than to complain. In some situations, though, the people telling their stories felt that there was no room for choice or change and that they just had to try to cope as best they could with the situation at hand. For example, the young man in "I'm the Full-Time Tenant of My Body" couldn't just get up and leave after his surgery when staff were not taking his complaints of pain seriously; he had to persist in trying to get the staff to listen to him.

One does not always have the energy required to challenge someone who has been inappropriate. The young woman in "The

Journey of the Green Elephant," for example, was advised to reserve her energy for getting well when she was tempted to lodge a complaint about the plastic surgeon who refused to treat her.

And sometimes it takes months or years to heal enough to truly find or reclaim one's voice or sense of self. Rachel Naomi Remen, in *Kitchen Table Wisdom*, says, "Somewhere along the way, our suffering subsides and our hearts begin to feel safe enough to open a little wider." The young mother in "When Loss Is Suppressed or Acknowledged" took twelve years to open up again and honor her first pregnancy. The wife in "Flying Blind in a Frightening World" waited for two years before she gathered the emotional fortitude to confront her husband's doctor and explain what she had needed. And the woman in "A Profoundly Isolating Experience" surfaced from her ten-year journey and sent a letter to her husband's hospital six months after he died; in this case, it tragically fell on deaf ears.

The Intensity of Memories

"What was the most touching moment during your time in the hospital?" provoked instant tears before the words could be formed.

"If you could say just one thing to a room full of medical and nursing students, what would you want to say?" stimulated a straightening of posture and lifting of a chin as the answer was spoken, with fierce conviction.

"What made your cancer treatment so positive?" evoked a smile of recollection.

No matter what questions were asked in the gathering of the stories for *Privileged Presence*, the answers were always clear and certain.

Health care experiences have an indelible quality. Whether a memory is fresh and new and only a week old, or is what one person called "twenty years mature," images, conversations (or lack thereof), small moments and gestures, and feelings of gratitude or frustration are imprinted on people's hearts and minds.

When our normal physical and mental functioning is uncertain, or when we are brought face to face with the fragility of life, all of our senses are heightened. As a result, health care experiences, for all the people who play a part in whatever the drama is, whether it be large or small, whether it be about birth or death, are situations that people remember with great intensity. How can it be anything but a privilege to be part of these moments?

Moving On

People who offered their stories for this book did so because they saw the value in having a collection of personal reflections about health care experiences. They understood that stories could gently provoke readers to think about what makes health care experiences positive or negative.

They also liked the idea of the wonderful company they would be able to keep with others who were coming forward to be part of *Privileged Presence*. Many discovered a sense of their own wisdom and courage as they voiced their stories and said it felt good to share their memories. One particularly poignant interview led to an unanticipated but positive outcome of the storyteller realizing she needed counseling to process her experience.

The storytellers in *Privileged Presence* are not alone. The momentum for change in health care is building. The movement is toward a new system of care in which relationships and communication matter. Increasingly, patients, families, and health care providers are finding innovative ways of working collaboratively and compassionately because they know they will achieve better clinical outcomes and improved cost-effectiveness.

It is comforting to know that so many people and organizations, in so many different ways, are working to improve the quality of health care experiences. Many of them are listed in the next chapter, "Building the Momentum for Change." Please get in touch with any and all of them. Find out what is happening, and offer your help and support.

> *"Never doubt that a small group of thoughtful,*
> *committed citizens can change the world; indeed,*
> *it is the only thing that ever has."*
> —Margaret Mead

Building the Momentum for Change

"How wonderful it is that nobody need wait a single
moment before starting to improve the world."
—*Anne Frank*

"I never lose an opportunity of urging a practical
beginning, however small, for it is wonderful how
often the mustard seed germinates and roots itself."
—*Florence Nightingale*

"We have a choice to use the gift of our life to make
the world a better place or not to bother."
—*Jane Goodall*

"I am only one; but still I am one. I cannot do
everything, but I can still do something. I will
not refuse to do something I can do."
—*Helen Keller*

Leading the Way: Key Organizations Committed to Developing Meaningful Partnerships with Patients and Families and Improving the Experience of Care

Institute for Patient- and Family-Centered Care

The Schwartz Center for Compassionate Healthcare

Canadian Foundation for Healthcare Improvement

National Partnership for Women & Families

Other Organizations Contributing to
the Momentum for Change

Useful Tools for Promoting Change

Patient- and Family-Centered Care:
Definition and Core Concepts

A Call for a More Compassionate Health Care System

Partners in Care—Conversation Starters:
A Tool to Facilitate Discussion

Key Questions to Ask

Better Together: Partnering with Families
Organizational Self-Assessment Survey

How to Conduct a "Walk-About" from
the Patient and Family Perspective

Educating Health Care Professionals

Sharing Personal and Professional Stories

Leading the Way

Key Organizations Committed to Developing Meaningful Partnerships with Patients and Families and Improving the Experience of Care

Institute for Patient- and Family-Centered Care

Founded in 1992 as a nonprofit organization in Bethesda, Maryland, the Institute for Patient- and Family-Centered Care (IPFCC) works to advance the understanding and practice of patient- and family-centered care in all settings where individuals and families receive health care and support.

Patient- and family-centered care redefines the relationships among patients, families, and health care professionals to create mutually beneficial partnerships. It encourages the sharing of information candidly and supportively. It fosters the active participation of patients and families in caregiving and decision making. With this approach to care, health care organizations and health care professionals invite patients and families to partner with them in quality improvement, patient safety efforts, facility design planning, in the selection and education of the next generation of health care professionals, and in research. (See page 320 for a definition and the core concepts of patient- and family-centered care.)

IPFCC is nationally and internationally recognized for its leadership in partnering with patients and families, promoting change in health care organizations, and enhancing the quality of the health care experience. IPFCC activities include:

* Convening in-depth seminars, *Moving Forward with Patient- and Family-Centered Care: Partnerships for Quality and Safety*, for interdisciplinary teams across the care continuum that include patient and family advisors

- Sponsoring international conferences that solicit presentations and papers from patients, families, clinicians, administrative leaders, educators, and researchers from the United States, Canada, and many other countries

- Offering webinars to further the understanding and practice of patient- and family-centered care

- Leading the campaign *Better Together: Partnering with Families* to change the concept of families as visitors to one where families and other care partners are respected as allies for quality and safety, essential to patients' health and well-being

- Developing and disseminating guidance publications such as *Changing the Concept of Families as Visitors: Supporting Family Presence and Participation*; *Creating Patient and Faculty Programs*, and *Advancing the Practice of Patient- and Family-Centered Care in Geriatrics*

- Producing videos such as *Partnerships with Families in Newborn Intensive Care . . . Enhancing Quality and Safety* and *Patient and Family Resource Centers: A Visual Journey*

- Publishing an e-newsletter entitled *Pinwheel Pages*

- Managing the website at www.ipfcc.org

- Hosting the PFAC Network, an online conversation and resource for anyone interested in the work of patient and family advisory councils and other collaborative efforts in all health care settings; participants range from patient and family advisors to health care staff, clinicians, and administrative leaders

- Providing on-site and off-site training and technical assistance to health systems, academic medical centers, community hospitals, primary care, and other ambulatory care clinics, agencies, and other health care organizations

IPFCC's website serves as an important resource on the evidence base and supporting literature for patient- and family-centered care. In addition, the site provides profiles of individuals and organizations that have implemented patient- and family-centered policies and practices. It also offers practical strategies and tools for how to advance this approach to care and how to create effective partnerships with patients and families to improve the experience of care and the quality, safety, and efficiency of health care.

IPFCC works collaboratively with many national organizations and agencies. A toolkit for hospital leaders, a policy statement and guidance publication for pediatricians, the development of an innovation community to improve chronic illness care, and multisite national quality improvement endeavors have resulted from these collaborative endeavors.

For further information about the resources and activities of IPFCC or about how to become involved, please visit www.ipfcc.org.

The Schwartz Center for Compassionate Healthcare

The Schwartz Center for Compassionate Healthcare is a national nonprofit organization dedicated to strengthening the relationship between patients and caregivers and preserving the human connection in health care. The center reflects the vision of Ken Schwartz, a Boston health care attorney who died of lung cancer at age forty and found that what mattered to him most was the compassionate care he received from his caregivers, which he said "made the unbearable bearable." He wrote about his experience in a now-famous article, "A Patient's Story," published in the *Boston Globe Magazine*. Ken founded the center in 1995—just days before his death—to ensure that all patients receive compassionate health care. The center is based at Massachusetts General Hospital in Boston where Ken received his care.

The Schwartz Center's signature program is Schwartz Center Rounds®, which allows doctors, nurses, and other caregivers to come together on a regular basis to discuss the most challenging emotional and social issues they face in caring for patients and families. The program has been adopted by more than 350 hospitals and other health care institutions across the United States and the United Kingdom and has been shown to enhance compassionate care, improve teamwork, and reduce caregiver stress and isolation. Issues discussed during Schwartz Center Rounds have also led to important changes in health care practices and policies to make them more compassionate and patient centered.

In addition to Schwartz Center Rounds, the center develops and funds other innovative programs, recognizes and honors outstanding caregivers, and works to make compassionate care a national health care priority. The center's goal is to ensure that compassion is a fundamental element in the design of health systems, the delivery of care, the measurement of quality, and the education of all health care professionals. Its *Call for a More Compassionate Healthcare System*, which outlines seven guiding commitments to advance compassionate care, is posted at www.committocompassion.org.

For more information about the center, please visit www.theschwartzcenter.org.

Canadian Foundation for Healthcare Improvement

The Canadian Foundation for Healthcare Improvement (CFHI) collaborates with decision makers to address difficult questions about how to organize, finance, manage, and deliver high-quality, affordable, patient- and family-centered health care for Canadians. Since September 2010, CFHI has supported seventeen teams across Canada who either involved patients and their families in decisions about service design and delivery or increased their capacity for more meaningful engagement in such decision making. Although the projects had diverse aims and used multiple strategies to engage their clients (e.g., advisory councils, surveys, and workshops), results demonstrate improvements to provider-patient communications (e.g., on pain management), the patient experience (e.g., increased understanding of emergency department care processes), as well as other quality domains, including efficiency (e.g., reduced mental health admission time from 4.3 hours to 1).

Lessons learned are shared through papers and webinars, and CFHI's online resource center compiles additional tools available to support patient and family engagement. Evaluating engagement activities is an important part of the program and helps participants better understand what works and what doesn't. For more information about the foundation, please visit www.cfhi-fcass.ca/whatwedo/patientengagement.aspx.

National Partnership for Women & Families

The National Partnership for Women & Families is one of the nation's most powerful and effective voices for women and families. It carries out its mission through focused activity in two broad areas: health care system reform and quality, as well as work and family issues. Engaging patients and families in system transformation is a central component of the organization's work.

The National Partnership is widely respected as an organization that works effectively with many stakeholders to build consensus and to develop systemic solutions that advance the common good. The organization has broad credibility, substantive policy expertise, strategic savvy, and access to the highest levels of policy makers, the media, and public and private sector leaders. Public officials frequently turn to the National Partnership as a key resource for developing policies that address the needs of patients and families.

For over three and a half decades, the National Partnership has profoundly impacted the systems and institutions of our society. The National Partnership won the landmark case that made sexual harassment illegal in 1977. It was a driving force behind the Pregnancy Discrimination Act of 1978. It wrote the Family and Medical Leave Act (FMLA) in 1984 and led the fight for passage until it became law in 1993. The National Partnership helped enact the groundbreaking Health Insurance Portability and Accountability Act of 1996 and the first federal protections against genetic discrimination, and led the multiyear campaign for the Patients' Bill of Rights. The organization also fought hard for key provisions to be included in the American Recovery and Reinvestment Act (2009), and the Affordable Care Act (2010) which significantly advance health care for women and families for decades to come. The National Partnership is known as an expert on issues related to the quality and delivery of health care services and the systemic changes that will be essential to moving to a better quality, more equitable, patient- and family-centered health care system.

Other Organizations Contributing to the Momentum for Change

Agency for Healthcare Research and Quality (AHRQ)
www.ahrq.gov

AHRQ funds, conducts, and disseminates research to improve the quality, safety, efficiency, and effectiveness of health care. AHRQ has made engaging patients and families in all stages of research projects a priority. Findings disseminated on the website assist all key stakeholders—patients, families, clinicians, leaders, purchasers, and policy makers— in making informed decisions. See the following links for further information:

♦ *Guide to Patient and Family Engagement in Hospital Quality and Safety*
   www.ahrq.gov/professionals/systems/hospital/ engagingfamilies/patfamilyengageguide/

♦ *Patient- and Family-Centered Innovation Series*
   www.innovations.ahrq.gov

♦ *Patient-Centered Medical Home Resource Center*
   www.pcmh.ahrq.gov/portal/server.pt/community/ pcmn_home/1483

American Academy for Communication in Healthcare (AACH)
www.aachonline.org

AACH serves as a leader in the research and teaching of relationship-centered health care communication. The organization offers in-person courses and conferences as well as online learning and publications.

American Hospital Association (AHA)

www.aha.org

The AHA is the premier membership organization for US hospitals and provides leadership and advocacy for member hospitals to improve care for patients and their families. Institute for Patient- and Family-Centered Care collaborated with AHA to develop the toolkit *Strategies for Leadership: Patient- and Family-Centered Care*, which is available for download at www.aha.org/aha/key_issues/patient_safety/resources/patientcenteredcare.html.

    Guidelines for the prestigious *American Hospital Association-McKesson Quest for Quality Prize®*, which recognizes a hospital with exemplary leadership aligning the agendas for quality, safety, and patient-and family-centered care are available at www.aha.org/about/awards/q4q/index.shtml.

The Beryl Institute

www.theberylinstitute.org

This membership organization is a community of practice for improving the patient experience in health care. It defines "the patient experience as the sum of all interactions, shaped by an organization's culture, that influence patient perceptions across the continuum of care." It offers a variety of in-person and virtual conferences, regional roundtables, publications, and other tools.

Caregiver Action Network (CAN)

www.caregiveraction.org

Formerly the National Family Caregivers Association, CAN is a family caregiver organization that works to improve the quality of life for those caring for others who are aged, disabled, or chronically ill. Their efforts seek to empower family caregivers, promote advocacy, provide peer support, educate, and provide resources—all for free and can be found on the website.

Center for Care Innovations (CCI)
www.careinnovations.org

CCI is a nonprofit organization, founded in 1999 as a collaborative endeavor between Tides and The California Endowment to foster innovation among safety net organizations in California. In 2013, CCI launched the *Engaging Patients to Improve Care* program to strengthen relationships among patients, families, and other members of the health care team and incorporate patient and family advisors in quality improvement efforts in California safety net clinics.

Center for Health Design
www.healthdesign.org

The Center for Health Design is a nonprofit research and advocacy organization of health care and design professionals who are leading the effort to improve health quality through architecture and design.

Center for Medical Home Improvement (CMHI)
www.medicalhomeimprovement.org

A "medical home" is a model for providing comprehensive primary care to children with special health care needs (CSHCN). The website has practical assessments and resources for providers in community practices and families serving on improvement teams. The complete *Medical Home Improvement Kit* including measurements, strategies, and *A Guide for Parent and Practice "Partners" Working to Build Medical Homes for CSHCN* can be downloaded from this site.

Childbirth Connection Programs
www.nationalpartnership.org

Formerly Childbirth Connection (and the Maternity Center Association), this organization has become a program within the National Partnership for Women & Families. Together they will advance the goals of better access, better care, and better outcomes. In 2014, they will release an issue brief, "Listening to Mothers: The Experiences of Pregnant Women in the Workplace," and an update of "The Rights of Childbearing Women."

Collaborative Family Healthcare Association (CFHA)
www.cfha.net

The mission of CFHA is to promote a comprehensive and cost effective model of health care delivery that integrates mind and body, individual and family, patients, providers, and communities. Educational resources, including selected articles from their journal, *Families, Systems, and Health*, can be found on the website.

The Eden Alternative
www.edenalt.com

The Eden Alternative™ is changing the experience of aging and disability. It seeks to eliminate loneliness, helplessness, and boredom by improving the well-being of elders and those who care for them by transforming the communities in which they work and live.

Emergency Nurses Association (ENA)
www.ena.org

The mission of ENA is to advocate for patient safety and excellence in emergency nursing practice. It offers a variety of educational programs and publications.

The Empowered Patient Coalition
www.empoweredpatientcoalition.org

This coalition is a consumer-led organization, reaching out to the public, to encourage and support their greater involvement in health care in order to prevent harm, enhance quality and safety, and bring about transformational change in health care delivery.

Improving Chronic Illness Care (ICIC)
www.improvingchroniccare.org

ICIC is a program located at the MacColl Center for Health Care Innovation within the Group Health Research Institute in Seattle, Washington. Its mission is helping the chronically ill through quality improvement and research. Its website provides resources about the Chronic Care Model, which views the patient as a partner with providers in decision making, participation in care, and quality improvement.

Institute for Healthcare Communication (IHC)
www.healthcarecomm.org

Formerly the Bayer Institute, this organization provides education and resources to promote partnerships between patients and providers in clinical practice. The website offers many resources for professional development including an *Annotated Bibliography for Clinician Patient Communication to Enhance Health Outcomes*, as well as case studies and training resources.

Institute for Healthcare Improvement (IHI)
www.ihi.org

IHI is a leader in advancing the improvement of health care. IHI's ever-expanding website has a wealth of information on patient and family involvement in quality improvement and research, including strategies to capture the patient and family experience of care as well as to involve patients and families on evaluation teams.

Institute of Medicine (IOM)
www.iom.edu

The IOM is affiliated with the National Academies of Science and serves as a nonprofit organization devoted to providing leadership on health care. IOM's major report, *Crossing the Quality Chasm: A New Health System for the 21st Century*, serves as a landmark publication in examining the problems of the current US health care system and offering strategies for change. Its 2012 publication, *Best Care at Lower Cost: The Path to Continuously Learning Health Care in America*, recommends: "Involve patients and families in decisions regarding health and health care, tailored to fit their preferences. Patients and families should be given the opportunity to be fully engaged participants at all levels, including individual care decisions, health system learning and improvement activities, and community-based interventions to promote health."

National Association of Emergency Medical Technicians (NAEMT)
www.naemt.org

NAEMT is an international membership organization representing emergency technicians, paramedics, and others working in emergency care. In 2000, NAEMT in partnership with the Emergency Medical Services for Children, published a series of documents on family-centered emergency care that is available online.

National Center for Medical Home Implementation (NCMHI)
www.medicalhomeinfo.org

NCMHI was created as a cooperative agreement between the Maternal and Child Health Bureau and the American Academy of Pediatrics. The mission of NCMHI is to ensure that all children with special health needs have access to a medical home. Resources, advocacy materials, technical assistance, and other tools for physicians, other staff, and families are available through the website.

National Patient Safety Foundation (NPSF)
www.npsf.org

With its mission to improve the safety and welfare of patients in the health care system, NPSF provides resources, including a specific area devoted solely to resources for patients and families who wish to get involved in patient safety initiatives.

Patient-Centered Primary Care Collaborative (PCPCC)
www.pcpcc.net

PCPCC works to ensure that primary care is the foundation of the health care system. It promotes the development of patient-centered medical homes, primary care settings in which partnerships among providers, patients, and families are central to the delivery of care and to primary care redesign.

Patient Decision Aids
www.ohri.ca/decisionaid/

This website is part of the Ottawa Health Research Institute and was created to assist clinicians and patients in working together to make difficult health care decisions. The program is research-based and the website offers online tools, clinician training programs, and other resources.

Patient Safety and Quality Healthcare (PSQH)
www.psqh.com

This online journal offers numerous articles highlighting the role of patients and families in patient safety and identifying strategies and benefits.

The Patient Voices Network
www.patientvoices.ca

This British Columbia network is a community of patients, families, caregivers, and others who wish to use their health care experiences for bringing about positive change. Members of the network believe that they bring valuable perspectives, insight, and experience that can be useful to leaders of health care organizations as they seek to improve patient and family experiences and enhance safety and quality.

The Patient Voices Programme
www.patientvoices.org.uk

This award-winning program was founded in 2003 in the United Kingdom by two individuals to facilitate the sharing of stories about the experience of health and social care as an education resource to improve care. Currently, there are more than 250 stories on the website.

Picker Institute Europe
www.pickereurope.org

Picker Institute Europe is committed to ensuring that the voices of patients inform quality improvement and health care redesign through measurement, improvement, and policy initiatives. Under the section entitled "Improving Patient Experience," Picker Institute Europe offers resources for partnering with patients and families in care and decision making and in efforts to improve the health care system.

Pioneer Network

www.pioneernetwork.net

The Pioneer Network is an umbrella organization working through advocacy, research, networking, and education to "change the culture of aging in the twenty-first century" and create care settings for older adults that are like homes and that are both consumer driven and person directed.

Planetree

www.planetree.org

A nonprofit organization based in Derby, Connecticut, Planetree seeks to develop and implement patient-centered care in healing environments. It provides information and education to all types of health care organizations, providers, and families.

Professionals with Personal Experience in Chronic Care (PPECC)

www.ppecc.org

A group of health care professionals established PPECC to advocate for improved systems of care after personal and family experiences with chronic illness and long-term care. Health care professionals are encouraged to share their personal experiences with the health care system in order to promote greatly needed change.

Samueli Institute

www.samueliinstitute.org

The Samueli Institute is a nonprofit organization supporting the research of healing processes and their role in health care delivery, with a commitment to transformational change of health care systems worldwide.

The Sorry Works! Coalition

www.sorryworks.net

This coalition composed of all stakeholder groups, including health care providers, lawyers, and patients, is promoting a transparent model of disclosure of medical errors titled "Sorry Works! Details" about the model, and related data are presented on the website.

World Health Organization (WHO) Patients for Patient Safety

www.who.int/patientsafety/patients_for_patient/en/

Patients for Patient Safety is a WHO program that fosters partnerships among patients, families, health care professionals, and others who have been affected by harm and who are dedicated to improving patient safety through meaningful collaboration.

◆ ◆ ◆

This list of organizations was prepared for the second edition of *Privileged Presence* as it went to press. Because there is such momentum for change, new organizations are emerging to participate in efforts to improve the experience of care. The Institute for Patient- and Family-Centered Care continually updates its website as positive changes occur. Please visit www.ipfcc.org for the most current resources.

Useful Tools for Promoting Change

Patient- and Family-Centered Care: Definition and Core Concepts

Patient- and family-centered care offers a framework and strategies to address many of the themes and issues in the stories presented in this book. By weaving the core concepts and practices of patient- and family-centered care into the infrastructure of every hospital, every emergency department, every clinic, every long-term care community, and every medical and nursing school and the schools for all the health professions, the quality, safety, and experience of care can be improved.

This definition and core concepts of patient- and family-centered care are presented as a resource for all those who would like to engage in improving health care.

Patient- and family-centered care is an approach to the planning, delivery, and evaluation of health care that is grounded in mutually beneficial partnerships among health care professionals, patients, and families. It redefines the relationships in health care.

Patient- and family-centered practitioners recognize the vital role that families play in ensuring the health and well-being of infants, children, adolescents, and family members of all ages. They acknowledge that emotional, social, and developmental support are integral components of health care. They promote the health and well-being of individuals and families and restore dignity and control to them.

Patient- and family-centered care is an approach to health care that shapes policies, programs, facility design, and day-to-day interactions of staff. It also leads to better health outcomes and wiser allocation of resources, and greater patient and family satisfaction.

Core concepts of patient- and family-centered care:

- **Dignity and respect.** Health care practitioners listen to and honor patient and family perspectives and choices. Patient and family knowledge, values, beliefs, and cultural backgrounds are incorporated into the planning and delivery of care.

- **Information sharing.** Health care practitioners communicate and share complete and unbiased information with patients and families in ways that are affirming and useful. Patients and families receive timely, complete, and accurate information in order to effectively participate in care and decision making.

- **Participation.** Patients and families are encouraged and supported in participating in care and decision making at the level they choose.

- **Collaboration**. Patients, families, health care practitioners, and hospital leaders collaborate in policy and program development, implementation, and evaluation; in health care facility design; and in professional education as well as in the delivery of care.

◆ ◆ ◆

Printed with permission from the Institute for Patient- and Family-Centered Care.

A Call for a More Compassionate Health Care System

*"In my new role as patient, I have learned that medicine is not
merely about performing tests or surgeries, or administering drugs.
These functions, as important as they are, are just the beginning.
For as skilled and knowledgeable as my caregivers are, what matters
most is that they have empathized with me in a way that gives me
hope and makes me feel like a human being, not just an illness."*

—Kenneth B. Schwartz (1954–1995)

If there is one issue that unites patients and their health care providers, it is the yearning for a deeper human connection. Compassion is recognizing the concerns, distress, and suffering of others and taking action to address them. As such, compassion is essential to high-quality health care and should be at the heart of our health care system.

Compassionate care is not separate from other kinds of care, nor is it reserved for the end of life; it is fundamental to all patient-caregiver relationships and interactions. Without it, care may be technically excellent but depersonalized and cannot address the unique cultures, concerns, distress, and suffering of patients and their families.

In today's health care system, we believe compassionate care is at significant risk. Despite improvements in quality and safety and a focus on patient-centered care, caregivers face numerous challenges that impede their ability to form meaningful relationships with patients and families, including fragmentation and uncoordinated care, burgeoning clerical and administrative responsibilities, increased cost and market pressures, inadequate reinforcement of communication and listening skills, and technologies that both help and hinder communication and relationship building.

To foster a more compassionate health care system, we are calling on all who believe in the importance of compassion and compassionate health care to support and endorse the following set of commitments, which we believe would go a long way toward making compassion a priority in our health care system.

1. Commitment to Compassionate Health Care Leadership

Health care leaders who embrace and model compassion foster a culture of compassion within their institutions and organizations. They play a crucial role in communicating the value and benefits of compassionate care and marshaling the resources necessary to make compassionate care possible.

2. Commitment to Teach Compassion

Health care leaders, educators, and caregivers who model, teach, and reinforce the core values and skills of compassionate care foster them in students and trainees. These skills include attentive listening, empathic concern, mindful self-awareness, effective communication, and the ability to elicit, understand, and appropriately respond to the concerns, distress, and suffering of patients and their families.

3. Commitment to Value and Reward Compassion

Health care institutions that value, support, and reward the cognitive, emotional, and collaborative work and time required for caregivers to provide compassionate care allow such care to thrive. These institutions are committed to the development of valid and reliable measures and methods to assess and reward compassionate care.

4. Commitment to Support Caregivers

Health care institutions that demonstrate compassion for caregivers equal to the compassion shown to patients and families help preserve caregivers' resilience and sense of purpose. Excessive workloads, lack of control, lack of rewards, loss of a sense of community with colleagues and co-workers, perceived unfairness and lack of respect, and conflict between organizational and individual values contribute to burnout and erode engagement with one's work.

5. Commitment to Involve, Educate, and Learn from Patients and Families

The needs and perspectives of patients and their families should be an organizing principle around which compassionate care is delivered. Patients and families should be involved in designing and evaluating care delivery and organizational policies at all levels. Health care, consumer, and advocacy organizations can play a key role in educating patients and family members about the elements and importance of compassionate care, their right to ask for it when it is absent, and to take action when its absence impacts their health or well-being.

6. Commitment to Build Compassion into the Fabric of Health Care

Those who design care processes should consider how changes in care delivery and associated tasks affect caregivers' capacity, ability, and time to interact directly with patients and families. The continuity of patient-caregiver relationships should also be a priority within and across health care settings as well as in the community to lessen patients' sense of being alone and unknown when they are most vulnerable.

7. Commitment to Deepening Our Understanding of Compassion

An integrated research agenda should be developed and funded to study the neuroscientific, psychological, and clinical aspects of compassionate care, its outcomes, and what compassionate care means to diverse patient populations.

◆ ◆ ◆

Please support our call to action and its seven guiding commitments by visiting www.committocompassion.org and pledging to do all that you can to ensure that our health care system is a humane and compassionate one for patients, families, and caregivers. The well-being of each and every one of us depends on it.

◆ ◆ ◆

Partners in Care—Conversation Starters: A Tool to Facilitate Discussion

When patients are asked to evaluate their health care experiences, common themes consistently emerge. Over and over, patients and their families say they want seven key things. These statements are listed following. They all evoke the same obvious question: "Are we meeting the stated priorities of patients and families?"

Use these statements as conversation starters in a variety of settings, from professional staff meetings and health care training classes to quality of care committees and health care planning sessions. Turn them into questions and ask yourselves: "How are we doing?" "Can we improve?"

- Patients want to be consistently and respectfully involved in decisions about their health care. They want their families involved in ways they choose.

- Families want to be consistently and respectfully involved in decisions about the health care of their family member.

- Patients and families want health care providers to listen to their observations and incorporate their preferences about treatment into the plan of care.

- Patients and families want and need useful and understandable information from health care providers.

- Patients and families want a personal connection, a relationship with health care providers. They need to be able to trust the people providing care.

- Patients' comfort and the control of their pain is important to their perceptions of the experience of care, and to their families' perceptions as well.

- Patients and families want information and support for handling transitions in health care.

◆ ◆ ◆

Printed with permission from the Institute for Patient- and Family-Centered Care.

Key Questions to Ask

Asking questions reveals what it is like to be in someone else's shoes. Asking questions is often the first step to understanding how one's health care organization is experienced and perceived by others. Leaders of hospitals, clinics, and community-based organizations should ask the following questions about their organization as part of efforts to improve and ensure the quality of care:

- Do the health care organization's vision, mission, and philosophy of care statements reflect the principles of patient- and family-centered care?

- Has *quality health care* been defined and does this definition include how patients and families will experience care?

- Does the facility and its signage create positive and welcoming impressions for patients and families?

- Are patients and families encouraged and supported to participate in care and decision making?

- Are policies, programs, and staff interactions consistent with the view that families are not "visitors," but, instead, allies for patient health, safety, and well-being?

- Are systems in place to ensure that patients and families have access to complete, unbiased, and useful information?

- Does the human resources system support and encourage the practice of patient- and family-centered care through initial interviews and orientation as well as ongoing education and evaluation practices?

- Do education programs prepare students and trainees for patient- and family-centered practice?

- ◆ Are patients and families involved in teaching students and trainees?
- ◆ Do patients and families serve as advisors to the hospital, clinic, or community-based practice?
- ◆ Do patients and families serve on key working committees such as quality, safety, patient/family education, and facility design planning?

　　　　　• • • • •

Note: This tool can also be used by patients and families. They may wish to share these questions with their health care provider or with the leadership of the organization where they receive health care. This gesture might begin a dialogue about how to improve the experience of care in ways that are beneficial to patients and families, clinicians, and health care organizations.

　　　　　◆ ◆ ◆

Printed with permission from the Institute for Patient- and Family-Centered Care.

Better Together: Partnering with Families Organizational Self-Assessment Survey

1. Does our hospital acknowledge the importance of families and other care partners to the care, comfort, and safety of patients:

   In written policies?

   In staff practices?

   On the website?

2. Does our hospital encourage patients to define their family or other care partner who will be involved in care and decision making, through:

   Written policies?

   Staff practices?

   Documentation systems?

3. Does our hospital encourage patients to identify their preferences for how family members and other care partners will be involved in care, care planning, decision making, in:

   Written policies?

   Staff practices?

   Documentation systems?

4. Does the hospital's family presence policy welcome siblings and children of all ages according to patient and family preferences?

5. Does our hospital make a distinction between *families* (as defined by the patient) and *visitors* (i.e., friends, colleagues, or distant relatives who may wish to visit), in:

   Written policies?

   Website?

   Staff practices?

6. Do our staff practices welcome families twenty-four hours a day and during:

    Rounds?

    Shift changes?

    Codes or other emergency situations?

7. Are patients and families welcomed as members of the health care team, according to patient preference, in information resources such as:

    Hospital website?

    Pre-admission materials?

    Patient/family handbooks?

    Unit welcome packets?

8. Does the hospital and its clinical areas welcome families through:

    Signage that is prominent and worded positively?

    Adequate and comfortable space at the bedside?

    Financial support for parking, if needed?

    Financial or other support for meals, if needed?

9. Is there a systematic process for gathering information about patient and family satisfaction with policies and practices related to family presence and participation?

10. Is the necessity of partnering with patients and their families as members of the health care team clearly addressed in:

    Orientation for:

      Clinicians?

      Other staff?

    Continuing education for:

      Clinicians?

      Other staff?

11. Is the necessity of partnering with patients and their families as members of the health care team clearly articulated in:

    Position descriptions?

    Performance appraisals?

12. Are there designated patient and family partners participating in the development, implementation, and evaluation of the hospital's family presence policy?

◆ ◆ ◆

Printed with permission from the Institute for Patient- and Family-Centered Care.

How to Conduct a "Walk-About" from the Patient and Family Perspective

One way to begin working with patients and families in planning for improvement is to explore your hospital, unit, or clinic through the eyes of patients and their families. A "walk-about" is an activity that can be used to obtain patient and family perspectives about the experience of care, especially about first impressions and how your organization's policies, practices, and environment support patients and families in engaging as key partners on their health care team.

If you have patient and family advisors working with your organization, ask them to participate in this activity. If you don't currently have any patients or families identified as advisors, invite several patients and families who have received care at your organization to participate. It is helpful to have more than one patient or family member participating in the "walk-about." Select patients and families who are willing to share their opinions. For guidance, see "Selecting, Preparing, and Supporting Patient and Family Advisors" in the resources titled, *Advancing the Practice of Patient- and Family-Centered Care in Hospitals: How to Get Started* and *Advancing the Practice of Patient- and Family-Centered Care in Primary Care and Other Ambulatory Settings: How to Get Started*, available at www.ipfcc.org/tools/downloads.html.

Instructions

Select a time when several members of the staff, as well as patients and families, can tour the facility together. It is helpful to have different disciplines represented. The tour should begin at the first point of entry into the hospital or facility (e.g., the parking lot) and continue to the inpatient unit and throughout the unit, including the patient room, treatment rooms, therapy areas, communication center and/or nursing station(s), family lounge, patient and family resource center, and other areas visible to patients and families. If this is an ambulatory facility, begin in the parking areas, enter the patient entrance, and follow the steps of a typical outpatient visit. Consider all the areas that patients and families may see or access.

You want to specifically explore how the following elements welcome, support, educate, and comfort patients and families and encourage their active participation in care and decision making. Pay particular attention to:

- How patients and families are greeted in reception areas, admitting offices, registration areas, clinics, and on specific inpatient units
- The processes of care and exchange of information with patients and families and among staff and clinicians
- Patient and family informational and educational materials for the ambulatory visit or a hospital stay and the transition to home and community care or different care setting
- Materials and information presented on bulletin boards, posters, announcements, and information kiosks
- Features that are encouraging and supportive of family presence and participation
- Characteristics of the physical environment (e.g., wayfinding, signage, artwork, color, lighting, access to views of nature, indoor/outdoor interfaces, visible equipment, adaptive features, and arrangement of furnishings)

The team should collect "evidence." Assign one or more members of the team to document the "walk-about" through:

- Digital photos or videos
- Notes from observations
- Samples of informational and educational materials
- Specific quotes or messages on posters or other announcements

Encourage patient and family advisors to share their perceptions throughout the "walk-about."

Although this exercise is designed mainly for staff to see the care experience through the eyes of patients and families, all team members should be given the opportunity to identify elements and processes that contribute to the experience of care and first impressions. These may be elements or processes that physicians and staff perceive as helping or hindering their ability to encourage patients and families to be active partners in care and decision making.

The "walk-about" activity can be a fun, nonthreatening way to begin to work with patient and family advisors and develop an appreciation for and level of comfort with the collaborative process. The "walk-about" can also be beneficial for patient and family advisors and potential advisors. It builds their understanding of staff and physician perspectives, care processes, and the environment of care. It allows them to begin to get a broader view of the positive elements of the system of care as well as areas for improvement. For new and potential advisors, the activity can build their interest and confidence level for serving as an advisor.

Set aside a meeting time to discuss what the team discovered through the "walk-about." Bring all the "evidence" to the meeting and discuss what team members learned about the experience of care through the eyes of patients and families. This tool can also be given to other staff to conduct their own "walk-about" to develop their ability see the clinic, unit, hospital, or organization from the perspective of patients and families.

The "walk-about" can be used as an initial step in the process of developing a vision, mission, or philosophy of care statement as part of a process to more fully integrate patient- and family-centered concepts and strategies in organizational policies, programs, and practices. It can also be used to develop a shared view of the current realities among administrative leaders, staff, clinicians, and patient and family advisors as a way to prepare them to "envision the ideal" and begin to plan and prioritize changes and improvements that will advance the practice of patient- and family-centered care.

◆ ◆ ◆

Printed with permission from the Institute for Patient- and Family-Centered Care.

Educating Health Care Professionals: Approaches for Developing Patient- and Family-Centered Knowledge, Skills, and Attitudes

The educational experience—undergraduate, graduate, and life-long learning opportunities—is critically important to shaping the practice and attitudes of health care professionals. This tool suggests content, teaching strategies, and support systems to integrate within curricula and the learning environment for students, trainees, and ongoing professional development programs.

In educational programs for physicians, nurses, social workers, and other health care professionals:

* Provide opportunities to listen to the real-life stories of patients and families and to have candid dialogue with them about their health care experiences and the implications for professional practice.

* Include experiential programs in which students and professionals-in-training:

  ▪ Spend time with patients and families in nonclinical settings such as visiting the home of a family caring for an individual with a chronic illness or life-threatening condition.

  ▪ Develop relationships with families served by hospital or clinic programs by working with the same families over time as part of assigned responsibilities.

  ▪ Attend a peer support or family-to-family support group meeting that is facilitated by the participants.

- ▪ Work in a variety of community settings providing health, education, and support services to patients and families.
- ◆ Provide multiple and continuing opportunities for students and professionals-in-training to work collaboratively with patients and families and with professionals from other disciplines, such as:
  - ▪ Attending a meeting of a hospital's patient and family advisory committee.
  - ▪ Serving on a multidisciplinary design planning committee that has patients and families as members.
  - ▪ Working on a task force with patients, families, and staff to develop patient/family educational materials.
  - ▪ Participating on a hospital-wide patient- and family-centered care steering committee.
  - ▪ Reviewing and responding to patient experience survey data.
- ◆ Integrate content on patient- and family-centered care when writing clinical textbooks and journal articles.
- ◆ Provide students and professionals-in-training with exemplary patient- and family-centered health professionals from a variety of disciplines as role models and mentors.
- ◆ Provide opportunities for reflective practice to enable students, trainees, and faculty to review and evaluate clinical, learning, and teaching experiences.
- ◆ Hire patients or other family members who have experienced hospital or clinic care as faculty and peer consultants for both clinical and academic programs.

- Model patient- and family-centered care and involve patients and families in discussion and decision making when conducting rounds.

- Require course work, reading, and discussion of patient and family narratives about the experience of care, the psychological ramifications of illness, and the importance of communication and collaboration.

- Honor the journey of becoming a caring, compassionate, and collaborative health care professional and provide a variety of options for personal support for students and professionals-in-training (i.e., peer mentor, faculty mentor, access to professional counseling).

- Provide continuing education opportunities for faculty and other staff to learn patient- and family-centered core concepts and skills.

◆ ◆ ◆

Printed with permission from the Institute for Patient- and Family-Centered Care.

Sharing Personal and Professional Stories

Many people have an intuitive understanding of the core concepts of patient- and family-centered care, but may not have applied them to their own health care experiences or their clinical practice. One way of opening this door to their own intuitive wisdom is through telling and listening to health care stories.

This exercise is designed to help participants develop an understanding of patient- and family-centered care by relating their own personal experiences to the core philosophical concepts (see below). This activity can work with any group but works best when the group is a mix of patients, families, and health care providers. It can also be used as part of the curriculum for students and trainees in the health professions.

Introduce the exercise. Explain that everyone is invited to think about and share a personal or professional story or experience that reflects patient- and family-centered care. Encourage people to share experiences that have created lasting impressions.

The stories should relate to the core concepts of patient- and family-centered care and can be positive or negative:

- Respect and dignity
- Information sharing
- Participation
- Collaboration

Personal examples might include someone's experience with childbirth, being admitted through the emergency room unaccompanied by a family member, or the hospitalization or death of a loved one. Professional work examples might include how a physician's initial negative perception of a patient changed over time or the way a nurse interacted with the brother of a young adult recently diagnosed with cancer.

Encourage everyone to share an experience, but be prepared that some people might not want to, given that this can be an emotional exercise. Offer to come back to them later or just let them "pass." They do not have to share a story if they are not comfortable doing so. Suggest that people be fairly brief—each person should take no more than two to three minutes to tell his or her story. You may have to be a gentle timekeeper.

If the group is large, you might want people to pair up and tell each other their stories and then, when the whole group convenes, ask for volunteers. This approach enables everyone to tell a story in a way that feels safe for those who may feel intimidated speaking in front of a large group.

During the exercise. Thank people for sharing as you go along. Occasionally link the stories back to the core concepts and point out how these stories help us see patient- and family-centered care from yet another perspective.

Conclusion. Ask participants what they learned from the exercise. Ask them how they might use what they learned in their lives or workplaces. Again, thank people for sharing their experiences. Let them know that stories touch people in long-lasting, significant ways. Encourage participants to use this exercise in other meetings related to patient- and family-centered care and to improving the quality of health care.

◆ ◆ ◆

Selected Bibliographies

Furthering the Process of Change

Stories and Storytelling

Furthering the Process of Change

The following bibliography includes written and audiovisual materials related to patient- and family-centered care and leadership to facilitate profound, transformational change in health care across all settings.

Abraham, M., Ahmann, E., & Dokken, D. (2013). *Words of advice: A guide for patient, family, and resident advisors.* Bethesda, MD. Institute for Patient- and Family-Centered Care.

Agency for Healthcare Research and Quality. (June 2013). *Guide to patient and family engagement in hospital quality and safety.* Retrieved from www.ahrq.gov/professionals/systems/hospital/engagingfamilies/patfamilyengageguide/.

Ahmann, E., Abraham, M. R., & Johnson, B. H. (2003). *Changing the concept of families as visitors: Supporting family presence and participation.* Bethesda, MD: Institute for Patient- and Family-Centered Care.

American Academy of Pediatrics, Committee on Hospital Care & Institute for Patient- and Family-Centered Care. (2012). Patient- and family-centered care and the pediatrician's role. *Pediatrics, 129*(2), 394–404.

American Association of Critical-Care Nurses. (2010). Family presence during resuscitation and invasive procedures (practice alert). Retrieved from www.aacn.org/wd/practice/content/family-presence-practice-alert.pcms.

American Association of Critical-Care Nurses. (2011). Family presence: Visitation in the adult ICU (practice alert). Retrieved from www.aacn.org/wd/practice/content/practicealerts/family-visitation-icu-practice-alert.pcms.

American Hospital Association 2012 Committee on Research. (2013). *Engaging health care users: A framework for healthy individuals and communities.* Chicago: American Hospital Association. Retrieved from www.aha.org/research/cor/engaging/index.shtml.

American Hospital Association. (2014). *2014 AHA McKesson Quest for Quality Prize Criteria.* Washington, DC: Author. Retrieved from www.aha.org/about/awards/q4q/index.shtml.

American Hospital Association and the Institute for Patient- and Family-Centered Care. (2004). *Patient- and Family-Centered Care Toolkit—*

Strategies for Leadership. Washington, DC: Author. Retrieved from www.aha.org/advocacy-issues/communicatingpts/pt-family-centered-care .shtml.

American Society for Healthcare Risk Management. (2010). Patient- and family-centered care: Making a good idea work {special issue}. *Journal of Healthcare Risk Management, 29*(4).

Berry, L. L., & Seltman, K. D. (2008). *Management lessons from Mayo Clinic.* New York: McGraw-Hill.

Berwick, Don. (2013). *Promising care: How we can rescue health care by improving it.* San Francisco: Jossey-Bass.

Blaylock, B. L., & Johnson, B. H. (2002). *Advancing the practice of patient- and family-centered geriatric care.* Bethesda, MD: Institute for Patient- and Family-Centered Care.

Blaylock, B. L., Ahmann, E., & Johnson, B. H. (2002). *Creating patient and family faculty programs.* Bethesda, MD: Institute for Patient- and Family-Centered Care.

Delbanco, T., Walker, J., Bell, S. K., Darer, J. D., Elmore, J. G., Farag, N., . . . Leveille, S. G. (2012). Inviting patients to read their doctors' notes: A quasiexperimental study and a look ahead, *Annals of Internal Medicine, 7,* 461–470.

Edgman-Levitan, S., Brady, C., & Howitt, P. (December 2013). *Partnering with patients, families, and communities for health: A global imperative. Report of the Patient and Family Engagement Working Group 2013.* Paper presented at the World Innovation Summit for Health, Doha, Qatar. Retrieved from www.wish-qatar.org/app/media/387.

Feinberg, L. (2012). Moving toward person- and family-centered care, *AARP Public Policy Institute, 1*–7.

Frampton, S., Gil, H., Guastello, S., Kinsey, J., Boudreau-Scott, D., Lepore, M., . . . Walden, P. M. (2010). *Long-term care improvement guide.* Derby, CT: Planetree, Inc. and Camden, ME: Picker Institute, Inc. Retrieved from: http://planetree.org/wp-content/uploads/2011/12/LTC-Improvement-Guide-For-Download.pdf.

Frampton, S., Gilpin, L., & Charmel, P. (2003). *Putting patients first: Designing and practicing patient-centered care.* San Francisco: Jossey-Bass.

Frampton, S., Guastello, S., Brady, C., Hale, M., Horowitz, S., Smith, S. B., & Stone, S. (2008). *Patient-centered improvement guide*. Derby, CT: Planetree, Inc. and Camden, ME: Picker Institute, Inc. Retrieved from http://planetree.org/wp-content/uploads/2012/01/patient-centered-care-improvement-guide-10-28-09-final.pdf.

Frazier, A., Frazier, H., & Warren, N. (2010). A discussion of family-centered care within the pediatric intensive care unit. *Critical Care Nursing Quarterly, 33*(1), 82–86.

Gawande, A. (2011). *The checklist manifesto: How to get things right*. New York: Picador.

Gerteis, M., Edgman-Levitan, S., Daley, J., & Delbanco, T. L. (eds.) (1993). *Through the patient's eyes: Understanding and promoting patient-centered care*. San Francisco: Jossey-Bass.

Griffin, T. (2010). Bringing change-of-shift report to the bedside: A patient- and family-centered approach. *Journal of Perinatal & Neonatal Nursing, 24*(4), 348–353.

Hardin, S. R., Bernhardt-Tindal, K., Hart, A., Stepp, A., & Henson, A. (2011). Critical-care visitation: The patients' perspective. *Dimensions of Critical Care Nursing, 30*(1), 53–61.

Hibbard, J. H., & Greene, J. (2013). What the evidence shows about patient activation: Better health outcomes and care experience; fewer data on costs. *Health Affairs, 32*(2), 207–214.

Hibbard, J., & Minniti, M. (2012). An evidence-based approach to engaging patients. In D. Nash, J. Clarke, A. Skoufalos, & M. Horowitz (eds.), *Health care quality: The clinician's primer* (pp. 245–262). Tampa, FL: American College of Physician Executives.

Institute of Medicine. (2001). *Crossing the quality chasm: A new health system for the 21st century*. Washington, DC: The National Academies Press.

Institute of Medicine. (2012). *Best care at lower cost: The path to continuously learning health care in America*. Washington, DC: The National Academies Press.

Institute for Patient- and Family-Centered Care. (2010). *Changing hospital "visiting" policies and practices: Supporting family presence and participation*. Retrieved from www.ipfcc.org/visiting.pdf.

Jabre, P., Belpomme, V., Azoulay, E., Jacob, L., Bertrand, L., Lapostolle, F., . . . Adnet, F. (2013). Family presence during cardiopulmonary resuscitation, *New England Journal of Medicine, 368,* 1008–1018.

Johnson, B. H. (2000). Family-centered care: Four decades of progress. *Families, Systems, and Health. 18*(2), 133–156.

Johnson B. H., & Abraham, M. R. (2012). *Partnering with patients, residents, and families: A resource for leaders of hospitals, ambulatory care settings, and long-term care communities.* Bethesda, MD: Institute for Patient- and Family-Centered Care.

Johnson, B., Abraham, M., Conway, J., Simmons, L., Edgman-Levitan, S., Sodomka, P., Schlucter, J., & Ford, D. (2008). *Partnering with patients and families to design a patient- and family-centered health care system: Recommendations and promising practices.* Bethesda, MD: Institute for Family-Centered Care. Retrieved from www.ipfcc.org/tools/downloads .html.

Josiah Macy Jr. Foundation. (January 17–20, 2013). *Transforming patient care: Aligning interprofessional education with clinical practice redesign. Conference Recommendations.* New York: Josiah Macy Jr. Foundation. Retrieved from http://macyfoundation.org/docs/macy_pubs/ transformingpatientcare_conferencerec.pdf.

Kenney, C.. (2008). *The best practice: How the new quality movement is transforming medicine.* New York: Public Affairs.

Leape, L., Berwick, D., Clancy, C. Conway, J. Gluck, P., Guest, J., . . . Isaac, T. (2009). Transforming healthcare: A safety imperative, *Quality and Safety in Health Care, 18,* 424–428.

Lucian Leape Roundtable on Consumer Engagement in Patient Safety (2014). *Safety is personal: Partnering with patients and families for the safest care.* Boston: Author.

Mattei, S. Y. (2012). *Sick, scared and separated from loved ones: A report on NYS hospital visiting policies and how patient-centered approaches can promote wellness and safer healthcare.* New York: New Yorkers for Patient & Family Empowerment and New York Public Interest Research Group. Retrieved from http://patientandfamily.org/educational-information/sick- scared-separated-from-loved-ones-hospital-visiting-policies.

Minniti, M., & Abraham, M. (2013). *Essential allies: Patient, family, and resident advisors; A guide for staff liaisons.* Bethesda, MD: Institute for Patient- and Family-Centered Care.

National Working Group on Evidence-Based Health Care. (August 2008). *The role of the patient/consumer in establishing a dynamic clinical research continuum: Models of patient/consumer inclusion.* Retrieved from www.evidencebasedhealthcare.org/.

Rittenmeyer, L., & Huffman, D. (2012). *How families and health care practitioners experience family presence during resuscitation and invasive procedures.* Joanna Briggs Institute, *10*(31), 1785–1882.

Ruder, D. B. (2006). Life lessons: Gravely ill patients teach medical students about listening and compassion. *Harvard Magazine, 108*(3) 44–51, 98–88.

Studer, Q: (2013). *A culture of high performance: Achieving higher quality at a lower cost.* Gulf Breeze, FL: Fire Starter.

Wen, L., & Kosowsky, J. (2012). *When doctors won't listen: How to avoid misdiagnosis and unnecessary tests.* London, England: St. Martin's Press.

Additional Resources

The Institute for Patient- and Family-Centered Care has posted bibliographies on twenty topics related to improving the experience of care; enhancing communication of patients, families, and health care professionals; and advancing the practice of patient- and family-centered care. These bibliographies are available at www.ipfcc.org/advance/supporting.html.

Stories and Storytelling

The collecting and sharing of stories helps health care providers develop a deeper understanding of patients' lives, their experience of care, and their context for disease, health, and wellness. As important as it is to honor the stories of patients and families, it is equally important to honor the stories of health care providers. Stories and storytelling are increasingly being used as an essential element of the education of health care professionals across all disciplines and in institutional efforts to improve the quality, safety, and experience of care. The following bibliography includes written and audiovisual materials related to stories and storytelling.

Aronson, L. (2013). "Good" patients and "difficult" patients—Rethinking our definitions. *New England Journal of Medicine, 369,* 796–797.

Callister, L. C. (2004). Making meaning: Women's birth narratives. *Journal of Obstetric, Gynecologic, and Neonatal Nursing, 33*(4), 508–518.

Casady, K. B. (ed.) (2009). *Caring: Making a difference one story at a time.* Pasadena, CA: Kaiser Permanente Southern California.

Charon, R. (2006). *Narrative medicine: Honoring the stories of illness.* New York: Oxford University Press.

Cohen, R. (2008). *Strong at the broken places: Voices of illness, a chorus of hope.* New York: HarperCollins.

CRICO (producer). (2006). *When things go wrong: Voices of patients and families* {DVD}. Retrieved from www.rmf.harvard.edu/clinician-resources/video/2011/when-things-go-wrong-film.

DeSalvo, L. (1999). *Writing as a way of healing: How telling stories transforms our lives.* Boston: Beacon Press.

Dickey, L. A., Truten, J., Gross, L. M., & Deitrick, L. M. (2011). Promotion of staff resiliency and interdisciplinary team cohesion through two small-group narrative exchange models designed to facilitate patient and family-centered care. *Journal of Communication in Healthcare, 4*(2), 126–138.

Dutton, K., Spencer, L., & Bennett, A. (eds.) (2011). *Connections—Nursing: Caring, Creating and Contributing.* Greenville, NC: Vidant Medical Center.

Epstein, F. (2003). *If I get to five: What children can teach us about courage and character.* New York: Henry Holt and Company.

Fadiman, A. (2012). *The spirit catches you and you fall down: A Hmong child, her American doctors, and the collision of two cultures.* New York: Farrar, Straus & Giroux.

Frank, A. W. (1995). *The wounded storyteller: Body, illness, and ethics.* Chicago: University of Chicago Press.

Gawande, A. (2007). *Better: A surgeon's notes on performance.* New York: Picador.

Gibson, R., & Singh, J. P. (2003). *Wall of silence: The untold story of the medical mistakes that kill and injure millions of Americans.* Washington, DC: LifeLine Press.

Gordon, S. (ed.) (2010). *When chicken soup isn't enough: Stories of nurses standing up for themselves, their patients and their profession.* Ithaca, New York: Cornell University Press.

Groopman, J. (2004). *Anatomy of hope: How people prevail in the face of illness.* New York: Random House.

Groopman, J. (2007). *How doctors think.* New York: Houghton Mifflin.

Gross, P., & Guersney, D. (ed.) (2010). *Pulse: The first year.* New York: Change in Healthcare Publishing.

The Healing Project. (2008). *Voices of caregiving: The healing companion: Stories for courage, comfort and strength.* New York: LaChance Publishing, LLC.

Hicock, L. (2004). *Beware the grieving warrior: A child's preventable death. A struggle for truth, healing and courage.* Toronto, Canada: ECW Press.

Hickox, S. (April 2002). Legacy of Angus. *Reader's Digest Canada Magazines Limited,* 171–198.

Jennings, S. (2002). *Locked in, locked out.* Saint John, Canada: Dreamcatcher.

Kabat-Zinn, J. (2005). *Coming to our senses: Healing ourselves and the world through mindfulness.* New York: Hyperion.

Kaminsky, L. (ed) (2012). *Writer, M.D.: The best contemporary fiction and nonfiction by doctors.* New York: Vintage Books.

Kenney, L. K., & van Pelt, R. A. (2005). To err is human; The need for trauma support is, too: A story of the power of patient/physician partnership after a sentinel event. *Patient Safety & Quality Healthcare,* January/February, 6, 8–9. Retrieved from www.psqh.com/janfeb05/ consumers.html.

King, S. (2009). *Josie's story: A mother's inspiring crusade to make medical care safe.* New York: Atlantic Monthly Press.

Kraft, D. (April 6, 2009). "Radiologist adds a human touch: Photos." *New York Times.* Retrieved from www.nytimes.com/2009/04/07/ health/07pati.html.

Larin, L. R. (ed.) (2013). *Inspired to change: Improving patient care one story at a time.* Chicago: Health Administration Press.

Manheimer, E. (2012). *Twelve patients: Life and death at Bellevue Hospital.* New York: Grand Central Publishing.

March, A. (2007). *Dying into grace: Mother and daughter . . . A dance of healing.* Cambridge, MA: Quantum Lens Press.

Martensen, R. (2008). *A life worth living.* New York: Farrar, Straus & Giroux.

McCullough, M. (2008). *My mother, your mother: Embracing "slow medicine," the compassionate approach to caring for your aged loved ones.* New York: HarperCollins.

Medically Induced Trauma Support Services. (producer). (2006). *The MITSS story* {DVD}. Retrieved from http://mitss.org.

Mullen, F., Fickles, E., & Rubin, K. (eds.) (2006). *Narrative matters: The power of the personal essay in health policy.* Baltimore, MD: Johns Hopkins University Press.

Nisker, J. (2008). *The other side of the fence: Stories from health care professionals.* Lawrencetown Beach, Canada: Pottersfield Press.

O'Kelly, K. (2006). *Chasing daylight: How my forthcoming death transformed my life.* New York: McGraw-Hill.

Patterson, J., & Friedman, H. (2008). *Against medical advice.* New York: Little, Brown.

Ratner, T. (2008). *Reflections on doctors: Nurses' stories about physicians and surgeons.* New York: Kaplan.

Remen, R. N. (1997). *Kitchen table wisdom: Stories that heal.* New York: Riverhead.

Remen, R. N. (2000). *My grandfather's blessings: Stories of strength, refuge, and belonging.* New York: Riverhead.

Rutledge, R., & Walker, T. (2010). *The healing circle: Integrating science, wisdom and compassion in reclaiming wholeness on the cancer journey.* Halifax, Canada: Healing and Cancer Foundation.

Schenk, D., & Churchill, L. R. (2012). *Healers: Extraordinary clinicians at work.* New York: Oxford University Press.

Schwalbe, W. (2012). *The end of your life book club.* New York: Alfred A. Knopf.

Shalof, T. (2004). *A nurse's story: Life, death and in-between in an intensive care unit.* Toronto, Canada: McLelland & Stewart.

Shalof, T. (2011). *Opening my heart: A journey from nurse to patient and back again.* Toronto, Canada: McLelland & Stewart.

Stein, M. (2007). *The lonely patient: How we experience illness.* New York: HarperCollins.

Sweeney, M. M. (1997). The value of a family-centered approach in the NICU and PICU: One family's perspective. *Pediatric Nursing, 23*(1), 64–66.

Taylor, J. B. (2008). *My stroke of insight: A brain scientist's personal journey.* New York: Viking.

Verghese, A. (1995). *My own country.* New York: Vintage Books.

Weber, D. (2012). *Immortal bird: A family memoir.* New York: Simon & Shuster.

Welch, J. R. (2012). As she lay dying: How I fought to stop medical errors from killing my mom. *Health Affairs, 31*(12), 2817–2820.

Williamson, C. (2010). *Towards the emancipation of patients: Patients' experiences and the patient movement.* Bristol, United Kingdom: The Policy Press.

Other Resources

Barron, R. (2012). *Twist of faith* {Kindle, iBook, Nook}. Retrieved from www.ridleybarron.com/store/.

Barron, R. (n.d.). *A victim's perspective on quality care* {DVD presentation, slideshow, and interview}. Retrieved from www.ridleybarron.com/store/.

The Examined Life Journal, a literary journal of the University of Iowa Carver College of Medicine. Retrieved from www.theexaminedlifejournal.blogspot.com.

Pulse: Voices from the Heart of Medicine, online personal accounts of illness and healing. Retrieved from www.pulsemagazine.org/email_guest_sub.cfm.

Index

Index

About the Authors

LIZ CROCKER'S career has included teaching, broadcasting, writing for newspapers, and running several businesses. She has held leadership positions with a number of health care organizations, including the Izaak Walton Killam Hospital, the Canadian Institute of Child Health, the Health Quality Council of the Province of Saskatchewan, and is vice president of the Institute for Patient- and Family-Centered Care. Liz co-owned a network of environmental stores for 22 years and has owned and run Canada's oldest children's bookstore since 1978.

BEV JOHNSON is the president and chief executive officer of the Institute for Patient- and Family-Centered Care in Bethesda, Maryland. She is a nurse and has been a trustee of several health care organizations. She has provided technical assistance to over 250 hospitals, health systems, primary care practices, and federal, state, and provincial agencies. She has collaborated with the American Hospital Association, American Academy of Pediatrics, American College of Physicians, National Partnership for Women & Families, and many other organizations to advance the practice of patient and family-centered care in North America and beyond.